What readers are saying . . .

'Thank you to Victoria for her honesty, her eloquence and bravery in this diary that has given me great courage. I was diagnosed with a form of Non-Hodgkin lymphoma in September this year at 43. [Victoria's book] normalised the chemotherapy process and debunked cancer myths while helping me in my recovery. You need to read this book.'   Simone from Ashford, Surrey

'I got the all clear on 6th October 2017. To celebrate I booked for my family to go New York. I read the book on the plane and was literally sat crying for the best part of the flight. Victoria totally sums up the highs and lows of having breast cancer. This book is a must read for anyone with the illness and going through treatment.'

Jo from Cumbria

'This book will give hope to women that are going through this disease, and help to the friends and family that are looking on.'

Linda from Basingstoke

'This really is a diary of hope and so much more ... So much of it resonated with me even though I'm living with a recurrence of a different cancer – the emotions and anxieties are similar irrespective of cancer type. ...by sharing her cancer experiences via her video diaries, Victoria has and continues to be continues to be a huge source of inspiration to others navigating similar.'   Jo from Harrogate

'I thoroughly enjoyed reading Victoria's account of her breast cancer experience having just finished my treatment at end of August. I would highly recommend it to anyone going through or having gone through the awful ordeal of breast cancer.'   Joanne from York

'This saved my mental health after my breast cancer diagnosis in June this year. The strength, confidence and hope this book has given me are so valuable'   Pika from Singapore

'This is a masterful, brilliant book. Victoria you should be employed by Macmillan as I have been too scared since diagnosis to open up any of the three tonnes of leaflets and booklets I have been handed!'

Online review

'By sharing her story, Victoria gave me knowledge and the comfort of not being alone. Even when you're surrounded by wonderful family and friends, it's only those who have gone through it themselves that can give you this. I recommend this book for anyone who has this illness or loves someone who does.'   Online review

'This book is without doubt one of the most touching and inspirational books I've read . . . It's a book that will give hope and support to anyone who has been touched by cancer.'   Online review

'If you only read one book a year (hopefully not!) then make it this one.'   Online review

'An amazing, courageous report of a journey through the treatment of this nasty disease. In sharing her experiences, she has given hope and helped many women facing the journey themselves.'

Online review

'. . . I've cried and laughed through a breathtakingly honest read.'

Online review

'Moving, insightful, warm, funny and poignant. If you've got cancer or know someone who has, this book will act as a valuable guide to getting through it. If you're fortunate enough to have never been touched by it – then it's a truly life affirming read.'   Online review

'An incredible account of an exceptionally personal experience . . . It is incredible to feel you have a friend that you have never met but in this book, that is exactly the feeling that you have.'   Online review

'An amazing courageous report of a journey through the treatment of this nasty disease. In sharing her experiences, she has given hope and helped many women facing the journey themselves.'   Online review

'As a reader I have laughed, cried and felt the anger as Victoria shares her thoughts, feelings and emotions in a beautiful, open and at times painful diary.'   Online review

Dear Cancer

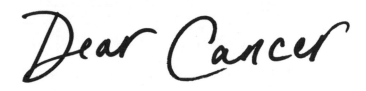

Dear Cancer

A diary of hope to
help you through

VICTORIA DERBYSHIRE

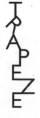

An Orion paperback

First published in Great Britain in 2017
by Trapeze
This paperback edition published in 2018
By Trapeze, an imprint of The Orion Group Ltd,
Carmelite House, 50 Victoria Embankment,
London EC4Y 0DZ

An Hachette UK company

1 3 5 7 9 10 8 6 4 2

A CIP catalogue record for this book is available
from the British Library.

ISBN (Paperback): 978 1 409 17296 3
ISBN (Export Trade Paperback): 978 1 409 17295 6

Typeset by Input Data Services Ltd, Somerset

Printed in Great Britain by Clays Ltd, St Ives plc

The Orion Publishing Group's policy is to use papers that
are natural, renewable and recyclable products and
made from wood grown in sustainable forests. The logging
and manufacturing processes are expected to conform to
the environmental regulations of the country of origin.

www.orionbooks.co.uk

To Joe, Oliver and Mark

Introduction

Over the years, many people have told me that when they first heard the words 'you have cancer', their mind went into a blur. Their fear was so overwhelming they couldn't take in any information afterwards, including the practicalities of treatment.

Now, when someone tells me that they've just heard they have cancer and don't know what to do, I wholeheartedly recommend this honest, engaging, and very practical book.

Through Victoria's experience, you get to see the day-to-day realities of going through cancer treatment: the endless drives to hospital for chemotherapy and radiotherapy, the sheer exhaustion that comes from having treatment. She also talks about the practicalities of looking after children, supporting a partner and working whilst being treated. And she shares what a breast scar looks like, and why she found losing her hair devastating. Most importantly, Victoria doesn't shy away from telling us that even with the best care and support in the world there are times when people with cancer are going to feel utterly alone.

Yet this is an uplifting book. We see how buoyed Victoria is by the love of her family and friends, the care of professionals and the kindness of strangers. She also gives us great hope by showing us that by taking it a day at a time and by knowing how to look after yourself both emotionally and practically, you can get through in one piece.

If you're a cancer professional, this book will give you a very clear idea of what your patients might have to go through, as well as how you might support them further.

If you have cancer, this honest and inspiring account from someone who has been there will be your guiding hand at the times when you need it the most.

Because we're all living longer and treatments are improving, one in two people born after 1960 will get a cancer diagnosis at some point in their life. Yet many people will speak about their diagnosis in hushed tones as there's still a taboo around it. I know that Victoria's generosity in sharing her experience in this timely book will give people affected by cancer – be it patients, loved ones or professionals – useful tools to deal with it in a better way.

Lynda Thomas
CEO Macmillan Cancer Support

Dear reader

I've been writing a diary since the age of nine. My desire to record what was going on around me may have been an early sign of my chosen profession, although I didn't realise it at the time. It was 1978. I'd never heard of the word 'reporter', let alone knew what one did; if you'd told me then that I'd end up working as a journalist for the BBC, there's no way I'd have believed you.

On Monday 23 January of that year, according to the entry in my pale blue Walt Disney diary with Donald Duck and Mickey Mouse on the front cover, 'I wrote to *Swap Shop*'. On Tuesday 24 January 1978, 'I posted the letter to *Swap Shop*'. What a year. (*Swap Shop*, by the way, was a hugely successful Saturday morning children's TV programme on the BBC.)

After documenting my primary school life on and off for those twelve months, it became a ritual – receive a diary for Christmas, start writing it on 1 January and keep going till the year ended. The teenage years were often about what I wore on a Friday night out, and not just a record of my blouses and pedal pushers, but what Leala, Rachel, Joanne, Andrea and Elizabeth were wearing too. It was the 1980s, after all. Plus, each Sunday evening I listed in my diary the Top Ten singles as I listened to the chart countdown on Radio 1. Waiting to discover what was Number One, live, *was* exciting.

And boys – there's loads about boys I fell in love with, particularly from 1982 to 1986 (Andrew V., Bim, Steve someone). Very occasionally I've filled a whole page with three words: 'Nothing happened today'. Sometimes so much happened, usually when I fancied someone or was at a gig, that I Sellotaped extra sheets of blank paper to the bottom of the page so I'd have space to write about every deliciously insignificant detail, folding the sheets neatly up inside when completed.

I don't read them, ever. I just have them, in chronological order, taking up a lot of space – tidily, though – in my wardrobe. There's something about having them that makes me feel . . . secure. A record, however imperfectly kept, of things I've done, people I've met, emotions I've experienced.

Yet I never expected to write in one of my diaries 'I have breast cancer'. Scribbling those words in black pen in my 2015 journal was brutal, devastating. Writing it down was confirmation that it really was happening to me. Suddenly this habit of diary-keeping I'd begun as a child became much more important to me, because recording the details of this unwanted experience gave me a semblance of control in my life at a time when control had been taken from me.

This book is based on my diaries from the summer of 2015 to the summer of 2016, documented in real time as events unfolded. When I read the entries back for the first time, I cried, because I'd forgotten or blanked out some details. The journals are pretty matter-of-fact because that's what I'm like, and most of my energy was focused on getting through the gruelling treatment that was going to save my life. I've used the diaries as a framework, adding in-depth reflections; I've included other bits too – letters, emails, cards and transcripts – which give an idea of what else was going on in my life and work during that time.

After one mastectomy, six sessions of chemotherapy and thirty doses of radiotherapy, the NHS staff told me there was 'no evidence of active cancer' left. I know I'm one of the lucky ones, and for that I'm exceptionally grateful. Yet many people now survive cancer – something you don't know when you're initially diagnosed. Then, in that moment, you automatically assume you're going to die.

That's one of the reasons there's a stigma around the illness. Conversations are often awkward or whispered because few dare ask if it's going to kill you, even if you happen to know the answer yourself. I knew I wanted to be open about having this disease; I wanted to show that you don't have to be timid when talking about cancer. We don't lower our voices if someone has Parkinson's, or dementia, so why should cancer have such power over us? It's an illness; the NHS treat it to the best of their abilities, and depending on your diagnosis, you'll deal with it, one way or another.

It's the reason I've written this book – to share my own experience. Not only to demystify the various treatments I endured, but also to let you know what the reality of having cancer was like for me. I found that, to my surprise, I could go to work sometimes, pick the children up from school, drink wine, all the while going through a strict treatment regimen. Not every element of my life had to be put on hold; something I didn't know until I got the disease.

This book is my account of how I approached my diagnosis and treatment. There are many ways to deal with both of those, and this is the way I did it. I'm not saying it's the right way. It's just my way. It's for every mum, daughter, sister, wife, brother, husband, dad and son whose life has been touched in some way by cancer. I hope it will give you strength and courage.

love
Victoria

Monday 27 July, 4.15 a.m.

The kettle's on, and I'm googling 'inverted nipple' before leaving for work. It's cautiously light outside, and it feels like it's going to be another hot day. Inside, the house is still. In order, this is what comes up:

Inverted nipple – Wikipedia

Inverted nipple – Embarrassing Bodies

Inverted nipple a sign of breast cancer? Doctor Answers [I could have clicked on this one but chose to continue scrolling down]

4 ways to get rid of inverted nipples

Inverted nipples – Go Ask Alice

And then I stop at 'Causes of Inverted Nipples – UK Health Centre'. This is what is written:

- Congenital – you may have simply been born with inverted nipples.
- Breastfeeding – this can damage milk ducts and make them more fibrous and retract, pulling the nipple inward.
- Surgery – scar tissue from previous surgeries may cause inversion.
- Breast cancer.

There are several more explanations, but I instantly stop reading. BREAST CANCER. At this moment, right now, in the early hours of this Monday morning in July, there is a profound shift in my life, from a lively, rewarding, ordered world of family, friends and work, to a world where I am no longer in control. Shit. SHIT. I might have cancer. I am not being dramatic, hysterical, irrational, foolish. I actually might have cancer.

Sitting at my kitchen table at dawn, quietly drinking a cup of tea with the blue light of the laptop reflecting on my face – it's a pretty mundane scene to accompany such potentially devastating news. Shall I keep googling to see if I can find another explanation? Shall I scream? I stare at the words on the screen as two thoughts overwhelm me: I don't want to miss seeing my boys, Oliver, eleven and Joe, eight, grow up; and, Mark and I should get married.

My mind races ahead: I can't bear not to be with these three most important people in my life. I can't bear not to be there alongside Mark as my children mature and flourish. My bright, funny, affectionate boys, who are never embarrassed to say 'love you, Mummy', and say it ten times a day.

My brain is being pretty smart. I know it's prohibiting me from formulating the words 'I don't want to die'. My brain is trying to shield me from something catastrophic.

I insist to myself that Mark and I are going to grow old together. But the reason 'we should get married' comes into my head is because I think I am going to be diagnosed with breast cancer and it will end my life, and so we should marry, in front of our two boys and Lizzi, Mark's daughter, who's twenty-two, with our closest family and dearest friends, and have a bloody great big party before I'm not there any more. I try to breathe at the same time as I try to work out what to do next.

Carefully I begin tapping out an email to Mark, who's slumbering peacefully upstairs, unaware of this shift in our lives. Try to keep things low-key by not using the word 'cancer' . . .

> hi darlin i noticed last night that one of my nipples appears to have 'inverted'; i have been feeling around it and it is hard. i've had a quick google this morning and i need to go to the docs.
>
> when u get up plse cld u call the docs and try and get an appointment for me this afternoon - when they say there are no appointments do say it is urgent (but i do need to see a woman plse)
>
> thankyou xx

I press send, and the noisy whoosh of the email flying off into the ether is far too upbeat for the message it carries. Then I leave for work.

At New Broadcasting House in London, I present our TV news programme in an efficient daze before going to meet Mark over at Radio 2, where he's producing music documentaries. In the summer holidays, he sometimes takes the boys in with him and then hands them over to me to take them back home. There's a tension between us; Mark's face is fixed with a frown and we can't smile at each other. Neither of us wants to address directly what I know we are both thinking ('what if I have breast cancer?'). He tells me he's made a GP appointment but that there's only a male doctor free. That's fine, of course. 'I am worried,' I say plaintively.

The boys are in great moods, not least because Zoë Ball has just nipped out of her studio at Radio 2 and seen Joe, shaken his hand and asked him if he's married yet. His blue eyes light up with joy and embarrassment under his long eyelashes. Oliver, Joe and I then go to an Italian restaurant for lunch, choose a table outside in the sun and I revel in their wonderful company. Tourists, workers and shoppers bustle by as the boys babble about nothing in particular, wind each other up and order lunch while I order breakfast. It's all so normal, except . . . I'm an observer, not a participant. I don't contribute; I want to absorb their chatter in a ridiculously intense way, because this really very ordinary lunchtime in our lives is suddenly a moment to cherish.

I'm at the doc's at 3.15 p.m. I explain to the children that I need a check-up on my right breast because it looks slightly odd. They happily tag along and sit patiently in the consulting room as I matter-of-factly give a short account to the doctor of what I discovered yesterday. I'm calm as I talk to the GP because I don't want to pass on any anxiety to the boys, but I can feel my heart pounding. His face is professionally passive as he informs me that an examination is needed, and we move into a tiny adjacent box room away from the children and a female GP pops in after I'm asked if I'd like a chaperone.

If you are looking at me straight on, as the GP is now, you will see that my right breast has collapsed; dropped an inch and a half lower than my left. The symmetry between the breasts is completely gone; as well as that, the nipple is being pulled back inward towards the breastbone. A tug of war between the breast and a tumour? Flat on my back, I stare at the greyish ceiling as the GP gently kneads around with his hands. And then – it's swift – within three minutes he softly announces he's referring me for an 'emergency appointment within two weeks for a mammo-gram and ultrasound'. We briefly lock eyes, understanding the significance of what he's just said. I get up from the bed, the windowless room suddenly not big enough for three adults. I feel short of breath, his words suffocating me, and I haven't even had a chance to put my bra back on by the time he tells me this devastating plan of action. I clutch my T-shirt to cover myself up before using it to dry my eyes as tears begin to flow. The second GP looks down, out of embarrassment or perhaps so there are fewer people watching me cry. Quietly distressed, I ask a series of questions but later can't remember what they were.

I ring Mark as soon as I get home, trying to remain vaguely upbeat. Why, I'm not sure. Make tea for the boys and wait for Mark to come back from work. Although I'm desperate to see him, when he arrives I can barely speak. That's not me at all. That's not *us* at all. I'm very open; I can talk about my emotions freely. Mark has become more open, particularly in the last few years, but there is nothing to say just now because we don't know anything for sure. No facts. And I'm not good without facts. There's too much we don't know yet to make conversation, or planning, possible. We sit in the garden in silence with a glass of wine each and our own thoughts. Eventually Mark tries to say something positive. 'We don't know it's going to be cancer.' In my head I say, 'We do.'

Tuesday 28 July

When the alarm goes off early for work and I remember the events of yesterday, three thoughts come into my head:

1. I feel like I don't want to breathe until I know if I have cancer.
2. I deeply regret cancelling our mortgage protection insurance at the start of this year because Mark will have to sell our house if anything happens to me.
3. I feel well.

Today's programme involves interviewing the new head of the National Police Chiefs' Council, Sara Thornton, about the changing priorities of the police when it comes to crime. My brain feels foggy and I find it almost impossible to absorb the brief I've been given ahead of her appearance. On air, though, I feel alert, managing to block out fears about my health, and the journalist part of me takes over. During our conversation, it becomes clear that Ms Thornton is arguing for police resources to be targeted towards crimes threatening the safety of children – sexual exploitation and grooming – and away from other offences. Bearing that in mind, I press her several times to be clear about where burglary would now come on her priority list.

Eventually, to be sure about what she actually means, I say, 'OK, it sounds like you're suggesting that if your iPad is burgled from your home, for example, the police might not come round and investigate?'

'It could be that,' she confirms.

I know her words will be picked up as a story everywhere online, and by plenty of tomorrow's newspapers.

After the programme, I sit outside BBC Broadcasting House in the sunny piazza and tell my friend and editor, Louisa Compton, why I've barely said a word to her in the last twenty-four hours.

'I think I might have breast cancer.' The tone is flat, numb. It's the first time I've said the words out loud, and they hang there for a moment.

She's taken aback. 'Jesus, why?'

I explain what's happened to the right side of my chest, and that the GP has referred me for an emergency appointment which will apparently happen within fourteen days.

Like me, she's a doer and her immediate reaction is, 'Why hang around for two weeks to see a consultant? Why don't I make you an appointment round the corner in Harley Street for tomorrow, and then you won't have this excruciating wait for information?' I don't feel that two weeks is actually very long, but Louisa plants a seed of impatience in my mind, and knowing that I'm always better at rationalising things when I have facts, I agree to let her make the appointment for me. When I arrive home, a letter from the NHS is waiting for me, informing me that I'm due to see a consultant called Mr M. Kothari at the breast cancer clinic at Ashford Hospital in Middlesex on 5 August. I had no idea until this moment that my local hospital even had a breast cancer clinic. This is becoming very real.

Wednesday 29 July

How is it possible to get up at 3.45 a.m., go to work, get your head round the morning's news, present a current affairs programme on TV, go home, mess about with your children, make the tea, watch/listen to the news, read all your briefing notes for the next day, go to bed and then actually *sleep*, when you think you might have cancer? I have no idea, but it seems to be the only thing I can do. Carry on as normal; because to disrupt the routine would give me time to think, and I don't want to have time to think further ahead than the next five minutes.

After presenting the programme I walk round to Harley Street, alone, for the 12.30 p.m. consultation with a GP. Just three days ago I noticed my right breast had collapsed, and now here I am, hoping against hope that someone will tell me it's not cancer. As it happens, she can tell me little except that I need a mammogram. Four hours later I'm having the first mammogram of my life, on both breasts, which essentially means squashing them flat into a large machine. It doesn't hurt, it's just slightly uncomfortable. Afterwards, I wait outside until the kindly lady comes back and tells me she needs to redo the procedure on the right side. 'Here we go,' I think.

It doesn't take her long to go away and scrutinise the second lot of images. I feel like I'm holding my breath until she comes back; when she does, it's to tell me I need an ultrasound examination. I'm ushered into a different clinical room and lie flat on a bed with a nurse to one side of me as a youthful, serious-looking radiologist strides in. He is calm and friendly; I am tense and friendly. The only ultrasounds I've had before were eight and eleven years earlier to monitor our unborn children. Then, I couldn't wait to strain my neck to see the image of the foetus growing inside me. This time I have absolutely no desire to look at what growth appears on his screen. As I look up, I see above me another greyish ceiling.

For several minutes he is silent as he concentrates. All I can hear is his regular breathing; all I can feel is the small oval device as he pushes it across my skin, revealing images of what's underneath. He's moving the ultrasound probe randomly: there is no pattern. Emotionally I'm shutting down for these excruciating seconds as I wait. Then he breaks the silence, bringing me back to reality, and describes what he is seeing as he starts to move the device in a more methodical manner, back and forth in the same area on my right breast. He's found something. His tone is low-key, his voice quiet and clear as he tells me he can see a 35 mm 'mass'. God. My mind scrambles to imagine how big 35 mm is – tiny, surely? How can it be a 'mass'? He says it isn't, though, a lump; it's more diverse, more disparate than that. More difficult to detect.

I am completely composed and focused because I'm good in a crisis, and this feels as though it's about to become a crisis. 'OK; what do you think I should do now?' The radiologist says I can have a biopsy there and then, or I can go away and think about it. I consider the options for thirty seconds and say let's do it now; at this point, and a little too hastily, I feel, the nurse asks me if I have private medical insurance. No, I don't, I'll pay for it on my credit card, I explain. The results of the biopsy will be back in forty-eight hours. That's fast. Good. I need information.

Thursday 30 July

I am completely distracted and can barely concentrate on work, but I know what's coming. I know I have breast cancer.

My close friend Cathy picks me up in the evening because we're having a chilled girls' night at hers. Her two boys and our two boys are great friends: they're the same ages, they all support West Ham and they met at primary school. Cathy and her husband Paul are diamonds. I answer the door, smiling and normal, I think, but as soon as we're in the car she asks me if everything's OK. She's picked up on a vibe, a not-quite-right expression on my face. I take a breath and tell her plainly that I might have breast cancer and should find out for sure tomorrow. She's shocked.

'Oh God, Victoria, oh my God, oh God.'

She says she knew something wasn't right as soon as I opened the door to her. She kindly suggests our boys stay at hers tonight so that Mark and I can simply concentrate on getting the biopsy results tomorrow. I gratefully accept, even though in my head I think I should be with Oliver and Joe at all times, in case that time is cut short.

Friday 31 July

We travel to Harley Street. It's a hot day, and I love London like this. Office workers are louchely draped around shaded squares eating their wraps and sushi. Suited blokes with sleeves rolled up are catching some rays in their lunch hour. But sitting in the waiting room even for a couple of minutes is too much, and I am starting to fret. The GP welcomes us into her office and I try to read her expression: impossible, because her face is impassive until we sit down, and then it changes to one of sympathy as she says exactly what I am expecting to hear: 'I have the results of the biopsy, and it is malignant.' At that moment it feels as though a colossal fist has come crashing down on my head, the word 'malignant' crushing me cleanly and swiftly. Mark captures my hand to hold it in his. My eyes are locked on the GP, who is saying these words in a compassionate, low-key way. She is waiting for me to react. I don't sob or swear – I am silent as I absorb her sentences and try to process what this means. The feeling of being battered lasts only seconds. It should take longer, but soon I am weirdly calm. And because I am composed, Mark is too. I am not afraid at all. After all, I was expecting this.

I react by asking dozens of questions (even if I wasn't a journalist I would do the same). I have an NHS appointment next week: will I get to see a consultant? What would the treatment involve? When will treatment begin? When will we know how bad it could be? And, importantly for me, is it wrong to try to compare this to some other illness – I can't think of an intelligent enough comparable example – but I know that what I'm already trying to do is make sense of it, and not give it a power it doesn't deserve. If I'd been diagnosed with diabetes, say, I'd be expecting to get on with being treated and I certainly wouldn't be thinking 'I'm *fighting* diabetes'. The GP seems to approve of this way of looking at it.

Mark and I walk out hand in hand into the sunshine of Cavendish Square in central London and find a bench. He hugs me very tightly and then my tears come. I say, it's unbelievable; it's outrageous; it's a fucking joke. I am cross and indignant – what the hell is going on? How dare this happen? And then there are no words as I cry into Mark's shoulder.

Once that outburst is done with, I move into practical, pragmatic mode. The speed with which my emotions switch doesn't surprise me. I don't want to dwell on it or analyse – I want to get on with it, and so we need a plan; I'm always better when I've come up with a plan, and we start to ring people. I speak to Louisa, who is shocked, supportive and kind. Mark rings a good friend of ours, Ben, who's a godfather to our older son, Oliver, and whose wife Natalie had breast cancer three years ago. They will know what to do.

I call Cathy; there's no reply. I call Cathy's husband, Paul, who's looking after our boys alongside his two boys, and tell him the doctor says the tumour I have is malignant, and is he OK looking after the kids until I meet them all at cricket coaching later? He manages to say, 'Oh God, Victoria, I am so sorry, we'll do whatever we can to help.' In one breath it's news of cancer; in another it's the everyday practicalities of getting on with life.

Mark goes back to work to sort a few things out, while I travel to meet Paul and Cathy at Chertsey Cricket Club. We sit by the side of the pitch while the children practise their batting and bowling. As I look out at my two running around without a care in the world, I have no idea how we're going to break this news to them.

Yet filling in Paul and Cathy, I surprise myself in that I feel pretty upbeat for someone who's just been diagnosed with cancer. Partly it's because at least I now know what is wrong with me. They both give me strength, and I tell them I'm aiming to be 'sorted' by Paul's fortieth birthday celebrations in November – it feels good to have a goal. Whether it's realistic or not I have no idea, but taking control of the timetable feels positive. Both are amazing, and promise they will be alongside our family every step of the way. Irish Catholic Cathy makes me laugh (first time in a few days): 'You just need to get the fecker out.'

I realise I won't be able to go to the Edinburgh TV Festival in a few weeks' time, where I'm supposed to be hosting a session. I email Guy Davies, a commissioning editor at Channel 5 who is organising it, to apologise and say I never, ever let people down when I've agreed to do something but on this occasion, I just have to. I don't say I have cancer; just that I have to have treatment for a condition that's been diagnosed today. He sends me a very kind and generous response as I realise that this is the start of trying to adapt my life around having cancer.

That evening, Natalie texts me and her words bring total reassurance that I am not alone: 'Hi Victoria, I know exactly how you are feeling right now . . .'

As I fall asleep (easily, as it happens), I consider the language most usually associated with cancer – military, warrior-type vocabulary that's not for me. I don't consider myself to be in a 'battle' with cancer, nor am I 'fighting' it. I just have it. And I want it gone.

Saturday 1 August

I wake, and for a few brief, light moments can't recall what's con-suming me. Mark is already up. Then I remember I have cancer (God, I've actually got cancer. Yet there isn't time to have cancer, I've got too much to do). It's officially my first day of living with this disease. To mark it, I go downstairs and announce to Mark as he sits at his computer, working, that I think we should get married, that I want to marry him but that I do *not* want him to marry me just because he feels sorry for me. He looks at me intently – Mark's been married before – pauses, then says with a completely straight face, 'I think marriage is overrated, to be honest.' It's a moment of black humour at a tense time, and it really makes us laugh.

My two bosses call me: Keith Blackmore, our managing editor, and James Harding, our director of news. They are wonderfully compassionate, ask several questions and offer total support. I say to Keith in an exasperated way, 'Can you fucking *believe* it?' I tell them I'm not depressed or frightened (and I don't think I'm in denial), I simply feel I have to be treated for this and then get on with the rest of my life. James asks if I've told my family yet. I explain I've already decided I need to see the consultant in four days' time so that I have as much information as it's possible to have before telling my mum, my brother and sister. At this stage there are too many unanswered questions, which would simply lead to anxiety. Plus, my sister's abroad with her family. Both tell me to do whatever I need to do to get well, in terms of time off work, and when I say I want to work as much as possible, they say they will be guided by me. James tells me he thinks my attitude is remarkable. I'm grateful to have such brilliant bosses.

Mark takes the boys out in the afternoon to see some non-league football, and I decide to read for the first time the pathology report I was given by the Harley Street GP yesterday. This is the document that details what's wrong with the tissue that was removed from me during the biopsy. I sit on the sofa, open my laptop and try to approach it like I would a brief for a complicated item coming up on the programme.

It's a mistake.

Cores from both the 10 o'clock and 11 o'clock lesions show portions of a grade 2 infiltrating lobular carcinoma (T3, P2, M1), with associated lobular carcinoma in situ. No vascular invasion is identified. Receptors to follow.

I begin googling to help me understand this terrifyingly in-comprehensible language.

It becomes clear that T3 is the size of the tumour (the smallest is T1); it's frustrating because I can't work out what P2 means, and does M1 mean it has moved or spread to other parts? It doesn't matter which website I use; I can't get a clear answer and the more I try, the more distressed I become. If it's spread, well then, that's it. I begin to wonder if I've been too optimistic, too confident. I hit a total lull and sob a lot. This is the first time I feel sorry for myself, and I really do, because I don't want cancer.

As I look up and around the sitting room, wondering what to do next, it strikes me that there are hardly any photos of me in the house, because I usually take the photos when we're out or on holiday. It suddenly becomes absolutely crucial that I rectify this, because, my thought process goes, at least if I die there will be some happy images of me in photo frames around our home. When people visit they'll point to my picture in a beautiful frame and ask my boys, 'Is that your mum?' I run upstairs and start searching. There appears to be only one where I look reasonable, so I put it in a spare frame and plonk it on the mantelpiece in the hall. That rather pathetic act seems to soothe me.

Ben and Natalie arrive that night and restore calm with their knowledge, practical advice and sheer upbeat attitude. It's a relief to talk to someone who's been through it, as Natalie has, and who's alive, happy and a picture of health.

We sit outside, food cooking on the barbecue, and fire questions at them both. What surgery did you have? What's chemo like? Did it make you sick? How long after a session of chemo before you were up and about? How much hair did you lose? Did you work through your treatment? How did Ben help? What can the bloke do? All the while the boys are playing on the trampoline at the bottom of the garden; each time they come over we change the subject because we aren't ready to tell them. Not yet; we still don't know enough.

Natalie explains what she experienced three years earlier: a Grade 2 breast cancer which had spread to some of her lymph nodes. (Grade 2 means the cells are growing at a moderate pace; Grade 1 is slow-growing; Grade 3 is faster-growing.) She had a lumpectomy (as it sounds – a lump removed from your breast, as opposed to your whole breast being removed), followed by chemotherapy and radiotherapy. In total, her whole treatment took around five months and her goal was being well enough to get back to work.

She tells me I have to take this a step at a time, and that even chemotherapy (if it comes to that for me) is doable. I remember Natalie wearing a fabulous wig after she lost her hair, and looking amazing. If I have to have chemo, then I will most likely lose my hair too. Ben reminds us that Natalie finally got so sick of bits of her hair falling out that she shaved it all off in the end. And there Natalie stops me – telling me not to think too far ahead and to take each part of the treatment in stages. It's exactly what I need to hear. They both make Mark and I feel optimistic again and, more importantly, back in control. They also advise me not to google incessantly, and to pick only one reputable website to consult *if* I feel the need to go online for information. They've given us a blueprint for dealing with this, and we are so incredibly grateful for their advice, support and positivity.

Sunday 2 August

A week ago, last Sunday morning, my right breast looked exactly the same as my left. I know that because I noticed nothing irregular when I had a bath first thing. By Sunday evening when undressing for bed, I did a double-take in the mirror. My chest had radically changed – the right didn't match the left any more. Grimly incongruous to think that a week ago I had cancer and didn't know it.

Monday 3 August

After work, I decide it's time to reveal a little more to the boys without telling them the full facts (not that I have the full facts myself yet). This is my rationale: if I gradually give them a bit more information, it'll make it easier when we eventually talk to them about the prognosis. So I introduce the subject of my body having changed.

I'm apprehensive, because the tone has to be right. Too much like an announcement, or too detailed or dramatic, and I worry that they'll worry and that I don't want. Employing a 'by the way' kind of style, I mention to them that there is something funny going on with my breasts. 'Funny ha ha? Do you mean someone's drawn a clown on them?' asks Joe. It soon evolves into a fabulously boysy conversation about the many different euphemisms for the word 'breast' – wibwabs, treasure chest, wop-bang-adula-do-wop-bang-do – which leads to uncontrollable laughter. God, I love boys. There is nothing as hilarious to them as a peculiar-sounding rude word, and that makes me happy. As a result, neither child expresses any concern or anxiety, which is my intention.

It's a beautiful afternoon, and we decide to go on a family outing to Cliveden House, where I take lots of selfies with Mark and the kids. Surreally, it feels like I am taking an official record of our day because it could be the last time I go on a day trip with them. Yet it isn't morbid. I can't help telling Mark, who kindly and firmly says, 'Don't be ridiculous.'

We roast a chicken for tea. I show Joe how to carve the meat. I know it's in case I don't have the chance to pass on the skills later.

Wednesday 5 August

I can't wait to see the consultant this morning – yes, can't wait – because he's going to be able to tell me if this cancer is going to kill me. As a journalist and now a cancer patient, I want the truth in order to confront it head-on. Mark, the boys and I troop into our local hospital, Ashford and St Peter's, bearing magazines, books and an iPad to pass the time; as it turns out, we sit around for one hour and ten minutes in the waiting room. It's large, square, pale pink (inevitably) and white, with rows of chairs facing each other, a bit like the seating arrangement in the House of Commons. There are no windows, no natural daylight, but it isn't miserable – it's bright and businesslike. Too bright – it's protesting too much. It's also extremely busy. I look around at the other women in there – perhaps twenty or so in total – some patients, some loved ones and friends supporting those patients. Their ages range from late twenties to seventies. I feel as though they look at me with particular sympathy because I have my children with me, but I could be wrong.

The boys stay outside when the consultant calls us in, shaking hands with Mark and me as he introduces himself as Manish Kothari. He is medium height, dark-haired with genial brown eyes; his manner is professional and serene. I gabble a little, and explain that I've already had a biopsy and have come armed with a CD of the ultrasound, a pathology report and one or two facts. He absorbs the information, maintaining eye contact throughout, and proceeds to ask me what I understand about my condition. 'I have a malignant tumour in my right breast,' is the simple reply. He asks to examine me and I move towards the bed as he draws the curtain around us. Mark is making notes – good advice from Ben – and a breast cancer nurse who's been introduced as Outra is also in the room with us. After the short examination, I put my shirt back on and sit down again.

Mr Kothari says this: 'I would recommend a mastectomy,' to which I reply in a steady voice and without a second's hesitation, 'OK.' He seems a little taken aback by how matter-of-fact I am, but I'm already there in my head: a mastectomy, yes, that's fine, when can we do it? We're due to go to Barcelona next week – please can we do it straight after that? I ask what the prognosis is, and am expecting him to tell me there and then whether I'm going to live or die. Patiently he explains that he can't answer that, as there are many more tests to complete before a prognosis can be made. I'm really frustrated. In my head, today is the day I'm going to find out if this disease will kill me. I don't want to wait any longer for that information; it's unbearable. But I'm going to have to.

Further tests include an MRI scan on the left breast and an ultrasound under my right arm to see if the cancer has spread to the lymph nodes (which I can have in the next hour, so that's something). The notion of the cancer having spread is chilling.

Outra is petite and pretty, with a warm smile, dark, shoulder-length wavy hair and her accent sounds . . . Caribbean? I can't quite place it. She leads us to a tiny room, where she gently talks through the various options for reconstructive surgery as a trainee nurse sits alongside her. She's not expecting me to make a decision there and then: it's more about explaining what's available. There are leaflets to look at, featuring images of implants, as well as actual implants – small, translucent, egg-shaped and rather pathetic-looking implants – for me to hold and squeeze. That's when my tears come – suddenly it's overwhelming. I am holding an implant which soon might be inside me because a malignant tumour and the rest of my breast are to be removed. I want information quickly, I'm impatient for it, but now it's too rapid and I can't process all that's been said to me in the last half-hour. Outra understands – how often must she have had this conversation in her time as a breast cancer nurse? Hundreds? Thousands? She stops and just lets me cry as I lean on Mark's shoulder.

Next, it's time for the ultrasound examination of my right armpit to see if the cancer has travelled to the lymph nodes. The ideal scenario is that it's only in my breast. While lying on the examination bed with Mark alongside me and the boys in the waiting room outside, I know I am trying to remain upbeat, even though I don't feel it. If it's spread, I think, that's it. The radiologist extracts some tissue with a needle from under my right arm (it's not painful) and immediately moves next door to check the cells under the microscope. While we wait, Mark and I barely say a word to each other. I'm just lying on the bed while Mark is holding my hand. She returns about seven minutes later to say this: 'The tissue isn't cancerous.' For us, it's such vital news, and yet she says it so calmly. My God, it's a moment of ecstasy (a 'champagne moment', Mark calls it), which totally transforms our outlook. For the first time today we are smiling, our hearts lifted, our spirits soaring. It means we can genuinely feel some relief, some joy, some gratitude – because things could be so much worse. Suddenly and determinedly, I know I can face this – I can do it, because I'm not going to die, not from this, anyway. And it will be fine. Mark points out that over the next few months there will be highs like the one we've just experienced and there will be tremendous lows – his job, on the advice of Ben, is to try to steer me between the two, along a more manageable path.

Leaving the hospital with the children, and buoyed by the news that it hasn't spread, we know we are going to tell them when get home; we know too that we are going to be totally honest and low-key with them. There is no way, we conclude, that we could keep this from them even if we wanted to (we don't). We cannot imagine trying to discuss this secretly, and them inadvertently finding out and potentially feeling betrayed that we hadn't been open with them. We've brought them up to be honest and to tell the truth, and now we want to do exactly that with them. That said, I do briefly raise with Mark the prospect of telling them without using the word 'cancer'. They know what it is, and I'm scared it will destabilise and even overwhelm them, even though they are pretty robust kids.

Mark points out that we've been straightforward with the boys about his depression (they understand the condition, know if he's going off to see a therapist) and asks, what if they find out another way? Hearing something at school, or someone coming to the door and giving me a big hug – or a bigger hug than usual – alarm bells would surely ring then? I agree, and call them into the kitchen.

Gathered round the island, we say we'd like to have a quick chat. I'm composed but slightly uneasy, because we simply don't know how they're going to react.

'So, guys' – I often call them 'guys'; it isn't an attempt to be all breezy – 'guess what?'

And then I slow down a little.

'It turns out that I have exactly what Natalie had – breast cancer.' I'm aware, in a broadcaster's way, that I give the word 'breast' exactly the same emphasis as 'cancer', so I don't make the second word sound worse.

There is silence, and the words hang there for several moments. Neither boy speaks. Joe looks down, possibly digesting what I've just said, but he might simply be looking down.

Painfully for me, I see a menacing shadow cross Oliver's face, and suddenly he is focused intently on what I'm saying.

I repeat it.

'So yeah, – maybe this sounds too casual – 'I've got what Natalie had – breast cancer.'

Pause.

'And we all saw her on Saturday, didn't we, and she's completely well now; and that's what I have. So . . . the doctors who we all met earlier at the hospital will treat me, and then I'll have surgery to remove a breast and then we can get on with our lives.'

Mark picks up the baton: 'And look at how well Natalie is. That's exactly how Mummy will look; and while she's having treatment, we'll all totally support her and muck in.'

Both boys are now looking at us. Neither asks any questions, which is very unusual for them. It could be because we've been too casual, or because they understand completely, or because they don't quite understand enough. Joe's expression is totally unworried, and by the end of my little speech, Oliver appears much less intense. We know it's gone reasonably well because they then ask if they can have a bit of computer time and they leave the kitchen.

I think they've handled it. I think.

My brain then turns to telling my mum, my younger brother Nick and even younger sister Alex. Alex is on holiday, so that will have to wait a few days, so I call Nick. If he lived round the corner I'd have told him face to face, but he's a couple of hours' drive away down the M4. I explain in practical terms, deliberately and without much emotion, what is going to happen. He is brilliantly supportive and very pragmatic and concludes with 'you can do this, Vic'. Calling my mum is much harder. She lives in Bolton, two hundred miles away, and again, this conversation would be better if we were together, but I need to tell her now. I begin with the 'hi, how are you?' bit and then go straight into, 'So listen, Ma, I'm going to be having some surgery in the next few weeks or so, because I have breast cancer; honestly, though, there is nothing to worry about, it's not going to kill me and I will be completely fine; it will just take a few months to get through treatment.' There is silence down the phone as she absorbs what I've told her. She is deeply shocked, and through tears says, 'It seems so unfair, so wrong; all you've ever done is work hard and look after your family.' I gently explain that more than one in three people* will get some kind of cancer in their lifetime, and that out of her three children it just happens to be me. It isn't 'unfair', it's just the way it is. She questions me about the diagnosis – I can tell she thinks I must be glossing over some bad stuff in order to protect her – but I insist that's simply not the case. She says she wishes it was her who had it instead of me, before offering to travel down immediately to help, but I

---

* The latest figures from Cancer Research UK suggest one in two will now get cancer at some point in their lifetime, partly because we're all living longer.

let her know there really is nothing to help with right now – in fact, I'm so optimistic about the diagnosis that I'm going to work tomorrow.

Thursday 6 August

When the alarm goes off at 3.45 a.m., I leap out of bed. It feels *so* good being able to go to work and present the programme. Louisa's abroad on holiday, but I've already emailed her to let her know I'm planning on letting our team know today. She agrees it's a good idea. In the debrief at 11 a.m. I ask if I can 'borrow' everyone for five minutes at midday for a quick chat.

Our team is a close-knit one, partly because most of us began working together at around the same time, back in March, on our brand-new programme. I want to be open with them about my diagnosis and be clear about the coming few months.

We gather near our desk on sofas, chairs, some standing, some crouching on the floor, about fifteen people in all, including our MD, Keith, who's come to support me. I deliberately choose to sit in the middle of Elaine Doran and Calum Macdonald. Elaine is a fantastic producer who worked with me on my old morning show on Radio 5 Live, and is now part of our TV team. As a teenager, Calum turned up at an outside broadcast we did in Edinburgh a few years ago with his dad because he loved our 5 Live programme so much and was desperate to get into radio. It's a source of pride to me that he's now making his own way in journalism.

I begin in a relatively clear, understated voice. 'I just wanted to have a really quick chat with you to let you all know that [deep breath] . . . I have breast cancer. It looks like I'll be having a mastectomy in the next few weeks or months. It's going to be fine. It won't affect the programme, and I'll work as much as I can, and the most important thing you can all do is to maintain the very high standards that you've set on the programme since we launched, and obviously email me work gossip when I'm recovering at home.' At this point I can feel my voice wavering and I see that a couple of the team, Julie and Katie, have tears in their eyes. 'I want to be totally open about the diagnosis. You don't have to speak about me in hushed tones, and you are not, under *any* circumstances, allowed to use the word "rollercoaster" at any point when we do talk about it.' Elaine chips in at this moment: 'Or "journey".' Laughter.

Afterwards, many of the team hug me, and later, they all send me wonderful emails, which I will keep forever. Today is a good day.

Louisa calls from her holiday and I fill her in about the team meeting. I also tell her I want to do something – reporting? writing? – to demystify the treatment around cancer. I'm vague about what I mean, but it's something I feel strongly about. It's partly the journalist in me, I suppose, but it's also because I'm learning what living with cancer involves, and because of the specific diagnosis I've been given, it feels less horrific than I might have expected.

At night, when Oliver's finished cleaning his teeth before bed, he asks a really good question.

'Are you not angry you've got cancer?'

I consider it, and tell him I'm not, because that would be a waste of my energy and I want to use all of it to get well, 'and anger is such a destructive emotion'.

As he gets into bed, he looks at me. 'Well, I'm angry you have cancer. I don't want you to have it.'

I tell him I completely understand his being cross, and that it's perfectly normal for him to feel that, but nothing is going to happen to me: I'm going to have some treatment and then I'll be well. And in a few months, it will all be over.

'So be angry if you need to be, and then let those feelings go. Let's concentrate on being positive.'

He accepts that, nods and I give him a huge hug before he settles down with a book. As I leave his room, I'm not distressed by this conversation, but proud of my son because he's been able to articulate what he's feeling.

Friday 7 August

On waking, I email a close friend of mine, Anna, to tell her the news.

Hi Anna

How are you? Hope you're okay ish and your dad is too.

Just wanted to let you know about some bloody boring news from me. I am having a mastectomy in the next few weeks because I've got breast cancer can you believe.

It's obviously shit but I'm being positive because at the moment, there's no reason not to be.

I'll call you later if that's okay.

I feel totally well and I'm in practical constructive mode.

What did we say about no more drama??!!!!

X

I'm due to have an MRI scan at St Peter's, Chertsey, the other half of the Ashford and St Peter's Hospital Trust. It's one of those where I lie on my back and I'm slowly shunted head first into a semi-claustrophobic tube. I've seen this on TV, so I feel fine about it. The scan is to check my other breast, the left side, for tumours. It is quick and the staff are efficient and professional. Every NHS staff member I meet so far introduces themselves and then takes time and care to explain the process I'm about to endure, always giving me an opportunity to ask anything I want to.

There's a letter waiting at home telling me my next appointment with the consultant isn't until 28 August. That's too far away. I want, *need* things to happen more quickly in order to get the information from today's scan so I can start processing it. I ring Outra, the breast cancer nurse, and also Mr Kothari's secretary to see if it's possible to bring the appointment forward. Outra leaves me a message later saying she knows when I'm back from holiday and that if an earlier time comes up, she'll slot me in.

As we stand at the moment, seven days on from a shock breast cancer diagnosis that I absolutely didn't see coming, this is doable. It really is. I'll have a mastectomy (or a double mastectomy if it comes to it). Then potentially I'll have chemotherapy as insurance to try to prevent any cancer coming back. And that should be it, shouldn't it?

I'm buoyed by my attitude. Then immediately doubt myself – am I in denial? Deluding myself? I know I'm not the sort to put a positive gloss on something when it's shit. So this, realistically, *is* how I feel. I can totally do it.

I ask Anna on the phone if she thinks I'm perpetrating a great big con trick on my brain about what I'm facing over the next few months. She doesn't think so (and she should know – we've been friends since our postgraduate journalism days in Preston twenty-five years ago). She is sympathetic and also wise. I talk through what I'm expecting to happen and when I can go back to work. Going back to the day job clearly represents normality for me, so it's a goal to focus on. I'm on leave for a bit, and after that it depends when the operation is scheduled for. Anna gently suggests spending more time with the boys and on enjoying our new puppy when we go and collect her. Several weeks ago, pre-cancer (that's how my life divides now – pre-cancer, post-cancer), we went to visit a litter of cocker spaniel puppies at a breeder's in Droitwich, and decided we definitely wanted one of the tiny black ones. We're due to collect her on 24 August, we've already named her Gracie and as a family we can't wait.

My pragmatic optimism is having an effect on Mark. He's normally funny, but at the moment he's making me laugh more than usual. Maybe it's a bit of a coping thing for him, but he's definitely trying to be as upbeat as possible around me. Suddenly, though, he says, 'Shall we cancel Gracie?' He raises it because he thinks he should, in case we're taking on too much. 'No way!'

I say. 'We're carrying on as normal.' Mark is delighted with my response, and agrees.

Saturday 8 August

I receive two gorgeous emails from members of the crew at work – Bex, our lovely floor manager, and Alison in Sound. I never expected such support from work colleagues, and it makes me appreciate even more what an amazing team we have.

I prepare to ring my sister, Alex, who arrives back from holiday this morning. It's important to work out what words to use and what tone to employ, so as not to make it sound over the top. I take a deep breath and call. When she answers, my voice is cheery as I ask how the break went, how her partner Alexis and her girls are, and she fills me in. We spend quite a bit of time chatting happily about the usual things, all the while wondering when I can change the subject in a non-conspicuous way.

'So listen, Al, I need to tell you something.' My voice is upbeat rather than dramatic. I plough on.

'I'm going to be having an operation soon because there are some cancerous cells in my right breast and they need to remove them.'

Pause.

Then Alex begins to cry, to sob. We are close, and I feel her pain because that's exactly how I would be if she was telling me she had breast cancer. My voice is steady as I tell her I'm not going to die, that having this treatment will help me stay alive and that it really is going to be OK. She's in shock, and I can't tell on the phone whether she believes my assertions about living. She asks various questions – how did I discover it, how bad is it, how am I, how long will it all take to be better – the usual, sensible questions that immediately crowd your mind when someone says they have cancer. By the end of the conversation I think (I hope) I've talked her round. It's clear that part of my job now is helping those around me who are overwhelmed with the news to stay positive, focus on the facts and banish unproductive worries. I'm happy with that responsibility.

Later I google Mr Kothari's name, and profiles come up under Bupa and a couple of private hospitals. Looking at his CV, what catches my attention is that he's a pioneer in 'nipple-preserving mastectomies'. Who knew that was even a thing?

Sunday 9 August

The kids and I watch Mark playing in a volleyball tournament in the sunshine. Later one of my oldest friends, Laurence, who I met working in BBC local radio in the 1990s, and his wife Rachel Corp (the editor of ITV News London) arrive to hear the details of my diagnosis and treatment. We shed tears because Rachel's sister Sarah is being treated for lung cancer (she's forty and has never smoked). We're drinking rosé, sitting in the garden and it's a special afternoon – sharing conversations and laughing – laughing in the face of shit, to be honest. Our human spirit amazes me.

Monday 10 August

I finally talk to Hayley in Edinburgh. We've been friends since we worked together at Radio 5 Live. I've been trying to get hold of her for a couple of days, and we keep missing each other. After a brief initial 'how are the kids?' conversation, I just tell her. 'So listen, Hayley, I've got breast cancer.'

'Oh, God, Victoria.'

'I know, I know, can you believe it? Cos I can't.'

In the post, a card arrives from Cathy, with the words POSI-TIVE THINKING printed on the front:

To our dear Victoria

We will be here with you every step of the way and available for any of the following:

– a hug

– a cry

– a shout

– a laugh

– a rant

And much more besides.

I've got some bloody good friends.

Tuesday 11 August

Today we leave for a week in Barcelona. It was booked ages ago, and we need it. I can't wait to spend time with Mark and the boys in a place that none of us has been to before. Mark has earmarked a bit of Picasso and Gaudí; the boys have already checked the fixtures at Camp Nou (as luck would have it, Barça are playing Athletic Bilbao in a cup game) and I'm looking forward to tapas and wine – oh, and forgetting that I have cancer.

Saturday 15 August

All week we've been impressed by the sight of holidaymakers hiring Segways and travelling up and down the promenade not far from our hotel.

The boys are really keen we try them, so after booking, we turn up at 5 p.m. for our lesson just as the sky starts to darken and glower. It looks like heavy rain is on the way. Riding a Segway appears simple enough, but Mark especially finds the braking part of the tutorial challenging and falls off about three times. It's why we're told to wear helmets. The boys and I are hysterical watching 6 ft 6 in Mark standing on top of a Segway, which makes him over seven foot tall, trying to tame it. As the storm clouds gather – real ones, not the ones in my head – we set off on our individual contraptions with me worried about the boys falling off and the instructor clearly worried that Mark will.

Ten or so minutes later, there's a public service announcement over tannoys to clear the beach as the wind really starts to get up, and we head back to our hotel. Our Segway teacher, no doubt relieved that Mark hasn't caused any structural damage to the Barcelona landscape, tells us we can finish our session another day when the weather's better.

A few hundred yards from the hotel, as spots of rain begin to fall, I start to get a bit cocky and increase the speed on my Segway, and suddenly my machine and I part company. I fall off, hit my head on the ground and call out in shock; Joe, who's slightly ahead of me, tries to jump off his Segway to help me. He too tumbles to the pavement and shouts out. At that moment Oliver looks back to see what the commotion is, loses his balance and hits the deck too.

The only one who doesn't actually fall off is the one you'd have put money on doing just that. Mark arrives slowly and steadily on his device to establish we're all OK, which we are; just a bit bruised and shocked. The instructor's concern is authentic, but you can tell he's relieved to say good night to us all, as by now he thinks we're a whole family's worth of liability.

Back in the hotel, we're hysterical again. Mark has christened us 'La Familia Penisio' because of our absurd collective clumsiness with the Segways (any play on words involving the word 'penis' really works with eight- and eleven-year-old boys). Yet suddenly a dark thought enters my head: did I black out just before I came off? I don't know the answer, but I can't be 100 per cent sure I fell off simply because of the rain and my speed.

Sunday 16 August

In order to miss the crowds, we head early for the park that Gaudí created, Güell. The pale ice-cream-coloured mosaic walkways, seats and fairy-tale gingerbread houses are absolutely stunning. As the boys run around, taking in every new artistic creation including the giant mosaic salamander, there's a moment when I wonder if this might be the last holiday I have with Mark, Oliver and Joe. Then I admonish myself because I detest morbid thoughts, but they pierce my mind when I'm least expecting it.

During the day I say things to the boys like, 'What kind of principles do you think I've passed on to you?' because I'm making sure they remember never to give up/be polite/always tell the truth, in case something happens to me. As we sit eating tapas in a lively outdoor restaurant at lunchtime, they must think some of the questions I'm asking them are absolutely bizarre, but I need to know the answers.

Later, by the pool, Mark and I have a conversation everyone should have when they're well – what do we want to *do* with our lives? After some discussion we realise it's taking our boys to all the places in the world that mean so much to us, if we can – Japan, Haiti, Montserrat, New York.

Astonishingly, cancer hardly intrudes on our holiday because I won't give it that power – although I do read Nick Robinson's book on the 2015 election and his cancer diagnosis. Mostly this break is like our others: a time when we take vivid pleasure in each other's company.

Wednesday 19 August

Back to reality. I am fragile today. The holiday's over, the next bit of life begins and I feel vulnerable.

While abroad, I received a lovely email from one of our sound guys, Dave, who told me he was shocked to hear my news and that he hopes to see me back in the studio soon because he reckons I'm a joy to work with each day. And an email from Shelagh Fogarty, too, which lifts me. Shelagh was a fellow presenter on Radio 5 Live, now hosting a daily show on LBC:

Oh Victoria

I am sooooooo sorry to hear that you are facing this.

Turns out I am really great with existential fear! You can immediately consider me part of Team Vic – I should warn you though, I might have T shirts printed.

You are a fighting girl (in the best sense) and I have benefited personally from that, so keep in close touch when you are ready for visitors or get Mark to be your envoy and give me a shout.

I'll keep you in my prayers too. I'm weird like that!

With love,

Shelagh xxx

Louisa arrives around 1 p.m. and cheers me up, filling me in with work gossip over several glasses of Prosecco (her) and rosé (me) at the kitchen table. In the middle of our conversation, erratically and randomly, I begin to cry. The tears are in charge, not me. And when they come I say, pathetically, 'I don't want to have breast cancer.'

She tells me the *Guardian* rang the BBC press office while I was on holiday saying they'd heard I was 'really ill'. I'm indignant because I'm not even a bit ill. It prompts us to discuss my writing something to put on Twitter, to let people know some facts and to explain to our audience why I'm going to have to take some time off over the next – I calculate how many – eight months? I can definitely do treatment for eight months, working out that I left Radio 5 Live in September 2014 and started our new programme in April 2015 – exactly eight months, and it flew by.

I know I want to be open about cancer, so now is as good a time as any.

Around 7.25 p.m., I post this:

Hi, have been diagnosed with breast cancer & am having a mastectomy in a few weeks. Family, friends, work & NHS staff are being brilliant 1/2

Will be doing the programme as much as possible during treatment in the months ahead 2/2

The very act of sending this message makes me think 'shit, it really is real', as though somehow it wasn't before. A piece of information I'd shared only with close family and work colleagues is now echoing around social media and there's no going back.

Within milliseconds messages begin to pour in, hundreds of

them, from all sorts of people I know and don't know: people who watch our programme, people who listened to me on the radio for years, women who've had breast cancer, women who are going through breast cancer treatment right now, men who've had breast (and other) cancer, men whose wives, girl-friends, sisters, mums have; colleagues, people I used to work with, people I hope to work with one day, journos, presenters, MPs from all parties, some of whom I've interviewed, some I haven't. One woman sends photos of a beautiful part of the country where she happens to be walking at the time, to cheer me up; several post pictures of themselves one year on, three years on, five years on from having had cancer, accompanied by words of wisdom, of kindness. It is overwhelming and brings tears to my eyes. People care and, oh my God, I cannot believe it.

Thursday 20 August

I wake up to the sun streaming through the shutters in our bedroom, check my phone and see that the sensitive, wonderful messages continue to arrive. It is astonishing to me that so many people are writing to me. A photograph of me is on the front page of the *Telegraph*, the *Daily Mail* and the *Mirror* (it's weird to *be* a story when my job is to cover stories). The headlines say I have breast cancer, aged forty-six. In this context it means I'm relatively young.

Richard Bacon rings – typical him, and I love him for this – not only does he want to hear the detail of the diagnosis and send me love, he also wants to talk about my tweet, the way I wrote it and the media reaction. I'm happy to indulge him. Richard and I worked alongside each other on the radio for years, but we became friends only after we left 5 Live. He says the messages I'm receiving on social media are restoring his faith in humanity.

I go to the hospital with Mark and we take the boys, who say they want to come along to support me. My heart bursts with pride to hear that. Today's appointment is for an ultrasound on my left breast to check the cancer isn't on that side too. The boys are fascinated by the technology and the radiologist, Demitrios Tzias from Greece, patiently explains how it works, as well as engaging in football chat with the boys (remember when Greece won the Euros?). Demitrios has a low, calm, reassuring voice – he'd sound terrific on the radio, I think. After the ultrasound he takes Mark and me next door to inspect the images with him as he talks us through them. We can all see a shadowy area at the front of the left breast just behind the nipple, which he suggests might need a biopsy. This news doesn't alarm me at all, because if it's cancerous, I think I'll have both breasts removed. If it keeps me well, I'll get rid of them. I ask if he knows whether I've 'caught it early'. It's a question various people have asked me. He says he cannot really know the answer to that – a cell could have been mutating for years.

'How long?'

'We cannot know for certain, but it could be up to eight years, or it could be much less than that.'

It occurs to me to mention to him that today, yesterday and once on holiday I'd felt dizzy, and there was the Segway incident

– did I black out before falling off? He pauses for a moment, thinks, looks at me and says, 'OK. In that case, I think you should have a full CT scan, which will check your body and your brain.'

It takes one heartbeat for that information to compute. At which point I say, 'Oh God.' It's the fact that Demitrios has specifically mentioned the brain.

There is silence.

The significance of what he has just said hangs there ready to swallow us up. We ask questions: if there's apparently no cancerous tissue in my lymph nodes (which there isn't), how is it possible that the cancer could have theoretically travelled to my brain? It is possible, he says; unusual but possible. It is an unutterably crushing thought.

We leave his room and walk purposefully away from where the boys are sitting. I'm pacing back and forth, my heart is beating fast and I'm panicking inside. I'm trying to process what is happening, and can't. Mark stops me and gently holds both my arms and tries to say something reassuring about the odds of it having travelled to my brain without passing through my lymph nodes being unbelievably low, and that this is something – another thing – we have to get through.

Within half an hour or so, I'm lying on a white bed that rolls back into the CT scan tube. It's claustrophobic, but that's the least of my worries. It takes ten minutes. Demitrios tells me before we leave that he'll try to let me know this afternoon what the result is.

Driving the short distance home, it feels like I'm suffocating. We pretend everything is normal to the boys. As soon as we're back, they go outside to play football and Mark and I sit opposite each other at the kitchen table. We have to talk about this, now; I can't tiptoe round it.

I take a deep breath and just say what's in my head.

'Darling, you might have to bring up the boys on your own. You may need to sell the house and use the money to live on,' I announce calmly. Mark looks visibly beaten down (and that's saying something for a 6-ft-6-in-tall bloke).

'We can't talk like this; it's not going to happen,' he pleads in a whisper.

'We have to. I know it's a nightmare, but it's going to help me – us – to plan; or at least, to talk about having a plan.' Although I'm completely composed, it feels as though it's happening to someone else, and I'm simply observing this kitchen table scene.

Mark can't or doesn't want to accept that we could be facing my cancer having spread and that I might not be around for as long as we'd like. I don't blame him in the slightest. But I need to confront this with him now, to be vaguely prepared, in control, in case the news from the hospital isn't good.

We discuss how much equity there is in the house, and how it would be possible to pay off the mortgage and downsize and potentially have just a tiny mortgage. It's surreal that I'm so utterly focused on the practicalities. It means there is no room in my brain to consider the cataclysmic emotional turmoil that we're now facing as a family.

Mark listens and barely says a word. He looks forlorn. I hug him and go upstairs to lie down for a bit while he cooks lunch for the boys.

After about forty-five minutes or so of me staring at the ceiling trying not to think about what might lie ahead, my mobile rings. It's Demitrios. Shit, this is it. I hold my breath, don't speak, simply listen. He's brief:

'Hello, Miss Derbyshire, I'm ringing to tell you your scan is clear . . . it has not spread to another part of your body.'

It's impossible to contain my elation, and I declare my affection and gratitude for Demitrios there and then.

'Oh my God, Demitrios, I LOVE YOU! Thank you SO much, thank you, thank you,' I shout.

I throw my phone on the bed, raise both my arms in the air, clench my fists and run downstairs screaming exuberantly to Mark, 'It hasn't spread! It's fine, he's just rung me and it hasn't spread.' The bear hug that Mark envelops me in is tight and shaking and joyous; it is without doubt one of the best moments of our lives.

This news buoys us so much, we feel as though we're invincible, and it gives me strength and confidence to face the treatment ahead with fortitude and positivity – because the alternative could have been so much worse. I am one of the lucky ones in the cancer lottery.

Our friend Juliet arrives back from holiday and calls immediately. She's got off the plane, checked her Facebook page and seen my news. She's subdued and concerned, but I tell her cheerily I'm not going to die, so there's nowt to worry about, and she perks up a bit.

Friday 21 August

I continue to receive many extraordinary messages, mostly from people I don't know. The feeling I have of deep gratitude towards those people is immense. Sentimental though it sounds, I feel as though I love them. Every act of kindness towards me, however simple or low-key, provokes an intense feeling of connection with the person responsible for the act of kindness.

Louisa alerts me to a piece in the *Telegraph* today headlined on the front page: 'Victoria Derbyshire – why all women owe her a debt of gratitude'. The thrust of Judith Woods's column is that by being open about the diagnosis I have, it encourages other women to check their breasts. I have no idea if her theory is true. The *Sunday Times*, *Hello* magazine, the *Daily Mail*, the *Observer*, the *Sun* and others contact Louisa and the press office at work to ask if I will do an interview with them. I turn all of them down, politely, because I don't want to do any. Perhaps because it feels too raw.

It's another beautiful hot day and we head to my sister's in north London to stay over. It's the first time I've seen her since my diagnosis. We hug a little longer than usual when we arrive. Her partner Alexis, who's a brilliant cook, hands me a purple clip folder which he's labelled 'Vic's Juices' (I must be ill – I don't even attempt some kind of double entendre), into which he's added various healthy fruit and vegetable drink recipes, like 'Super Orange Booster – pre-surgery', and 'Green Spinach & Pear Juice – post-surgery convalescence'. He also gives me a juicer. Such a simple, thoughtful gesture makes me cry – Alex confesses that when he initially showed it to her, she cried too. I think it's good for my sister to see me, and to see that I'm fine, physically and mentally. Mark joins us after work and we drink and eat in a very happy atmosphere. None of us is morbid in the slightest.

Saturday 22 August

On a walk in the local park the next morning with all the kids, Alex and I discuss the pros and cons of reconstructive surgery. I'm not an expert in this area (clearly), but I try to explain that the consultant, Mr Kothari, is planning to carry out a 'nipple-preserving mastectomy'. That means cutting just under the bottom part of the right breast, lifting up the skin, removing the tumour and any other cancerous cells, inserting an implant, drawing the skin back over the implant and sewing it up underneath. I discuss my reservations about having an implant – not for safety reasons: I know these ones are safe – but it's the idea of having something false, something artificial inside me. I also think I wouldn't mind being flat on one side with a scar. But then, as Alex points out, whenever you put a bra on you'd have to insert some kind of filling to balance out your bra underneath your clothing.

As we leave, Alexis hands us a home-made moussaka and several portions of Bolognese sauce which we can put in the freezer. He is one thoughtful dude, and we truly appreciate this kind of practical gesture.

On arriving home, there are pretty flowers on the doorstep

from our ex-neighbours, lovely Julian and Christine, a card from our current neighbours Guy and Louise with a note offering help with anything, a gift from Hayley (a state-of-the-art juicer; seriously, you wait all your life for a juicer and two come along at once), as well as a marvellous card from a woman I've never met who lives in our village:

Dear Victoria

Please forgive me for being intrusive as we don't know one another. I live in the village and last Thursday had a double mastectomy under Ashford & St Peter's Hospital and I would like to say how amazing the breast care team have been. I'm a week into my recovery and heard your news on breakfast TV and wanted to reach out to you as I can imagine how you're feeling having just been diagnosed myself. If I can be of any help with any questions, or answer any of your fears, please call me if you wish to. I would like to wish you the very best in your forthcoming treatment. Take care, Victoria.

Yours,

Jill

How compassionate is that? She's written her number on the card, and I text her immediately to thank her for extending the hand of friendship and also because I'm eager to ask questions of someone who's been through what lies ahead of me. We arrange for me to visit her next week. I can't wait. Information is what I need to keep me rational and buoyant.

Sunday 23 August

I am spending much of today trying to reply to or favourite all the messages I continue to receive from people on Facebook and Twitter. It's important to me that I acknowledge as many people as I can, because I want each one to know how much their sensible, sympathetic words mean to me.

Monday 24 August

Mark, Oliver, Joe and I go to pick up our puppy, Gracie, from the breeder's to bring her back to her new home. When we see her again after a gap of six or seven weeks, we can't believe how beautiful she is. Her black shiny body fits into Mark's hand, and she clambers up to his face to lick his stubble. The boys cup her in their hands and pull her to their chests. She is adorable. Gracie sits on my lap all the way home from the Midlands to London and cries a little, but as soon as she arrives at our house she races into the garden and straight into some flowers. What a delicious bundle of joy. Just what we need as a family right now.

Tuesday 25 August

Well, Gracie didn't cry at all last night, which we'd been warned to expect. She is amazing, and seems to be very happy.

I ring Outra – still no appointment at Harrow for a biopsy on the left breast, but she says she's trying to get one for tomorrow morning. I feel impatient, but there's little I can do to speed things up.

On the way to visit my new-found neighbour Jill, a five-minute walk up the river, Ceri Thomas rings me, my former editor on Radio 5 Live *Breakfast*, now at *Panorama* via Radio 4's *Today* programme. It's an upbeat, matter-of-fact conversation along the lines of:

Me: 'Can you fucking believe it, Ceri?! What the fuck is going on?'

Him: [laughter] 'It *is* unbelievable, but you've just gotta get on with it.'

Me: 'I know, I know, I'm already there, I know that, I've just gotta get through it and crack on.'

I'm happy (and nervous) to be seeing Jill, because I'm hoping she'll be able to give me answers to questions such as: how long does it take to recover from a mastectomy? When can you go back to work? When can you drive again? All my worries are practical, and I know that as soon as I have those answers, I can really plan and work out my timescale of recovery. I decide to take with me a card and some pink champagne as a gift. Jill opens her front door and I immediately feel a warmth from her as a kindred spirit. She's fifty, has blonde hair and a friendly face and my nerves disappear immediately. She also has a dog, Benji, a golden doodle (golden retriever mixed with a standard poodle). At this point I know I'm going to get on with her, and I tell her all about the new canine addition to our family.

While the kettle's on, she explains she'd been watching Lorraine Kelly's programme last week, and Lorraine had talked about my diagnosis and wished me all the best. Lorraine had then read out my tweet on air which mentioned the NHS, and this resourceful lady Jill, knowing I lived in the same village, worked out that I must be being treated at the same hospital as her. (I did the newspaper review on Lorraine's programme for about three years, and she sent me a very compassionate direct message on Twitter last Thursday.)

Jill tells me about her double mastectomy, that she's in her second week of recovery and that her mum and grandma both died of breast cancer. At this point tears start to flow down my face without my being able to stop them as I say, 'Oh God, I am so sorry.' Jill ends up comforting me, which is the wrong way round, adding that it was a long time ago but that her two grown-up daughters will have to be tested for the gene at some point. We talk intently for two hours.

'Do you want to see my drains?'

'Your what?' I ask, bemused. I have no idea what she's talking about, but suspect it's nothing to do with her domestic plumbing arrangements.

'My drains – the things that drain the fluid from your breasts after the surgery.'

It sounds grim – both the word itself and the practicalities. They don't look that elegant, either: two half-metre plastic tubes protrude from each side of Jill's breasts, at the end of which is a round plastic ball which collects – as far as I can see – blood. Jill's cleverly hidden most of the tubes and balls in a small handbag she wears diagonally across her body. They are pretty revolting, hardly dignified but discreet enough, I think, not to be a problem or inhibit me going out. I certainly hadn't noticed four hollow cylinders sticking out of Jill when I arrived.

Before I leave she asks if I would like to see her scars, what the aftermath of a double mastectomy looks like. I consider this for a few seconds and surprise myself by saying no. Although I'm hugely curious, of course, I don't feel ready. I thank her profusely for her time, wish her luck in her continued recovery and we promise to keep in touch.

The afternoon is spent doing jobs – picking up Oliver's school uniform for his new secondary school, going to a Pilates class and doing a bit of food shopping. Life has to go on, even during cancer.

At night, Mark and the boys take Gracie for her first puppy training class. She's a delight – a 'superdog', I call her. Once she's ready, I could take her for a walk with Jill and Benji.

Wednesday 26 August

It's exactly one month since my breast collapsed. In that time I've learned I have cancer, that I'm about to have life-saving surgery, that I couldn't do this without my family and friends, and that astonishing kindness from complete strangers is lifting my spirits no end. I also realise that at this moment, the negatives of having cancer aren't outweighing the positives. If 'negative' and 'positive' were placed on Lady Justice's scales, they would be of equal weight. I don't want this illness, but as I have no choice, it's gratifying that there are so many things to cheer me.

Mark and I leave the house at 7 a.m. to drive to Northwick Park Hospital in Harrow for an 8 a.m. appointment to have a biopsy on my left breast. The boys are left in charge of Gracie, with clear instructions to encourage her constantly into the garden to do a wee. They are apprehensive and also delighted with the responsibility, although Oliver isn't particularly enamoured with the prospect of clearing up any poo in the garden.

There's loads of traffic, and I am starting to feel stressed about us missing the appointment. I hate being late for anything (a by-product of my mum being late for everything when we were kids, so I'm now the opposite), but being late for something like this, which will take me a step further down the road of being well again, makes me very tense.

As it happens we're on time, and soon a consultant called Dr Morgan is introducing herself to us. She's young, slim, professional and serious, and carefully explains how the biopsy will work: I will remove the clothing from my top half and lie on my front on a hard bed that has two concave holes where, effectively, my breasts will sit. With precise measurements, and after an anaesthetic in my left side, a needle will be inserted into my flesh in order to remove some tissue, which will then be examined.

Another member of staff helps me get into the right position on the bed, and I ask her name and where she's from – she's Bromiley from Nepal. I make a mental note that, if I remember, I'd like to collect the names of everyone who treats me and where they're from.

Because of the anaesthetic, the biopsy itself is painless. As I'm extracting myself from the bed, Dr Morgan tells me not to look down, which of course I do immediately, and see quite a bit of blood and tissue spattered beneath me. Although it looks pretty gruesome it doesn't bother me, because everything that's being done now is to collect more information. Once the medics have all the facts they need, they can get on with the treatment.

I feel upbeat as we leave, telling Mark that if the results of this biopsy suggest there are cancerous cells in the left side, then I'll simply have a double mastectomy. I email Louisa the same info. If it's good enough for Angelina, it's good enough for me.

In the evening, I give Mark a card thanking him for being brilliant – calm, kind and very sensible.

Thursday 27 August

On a daily basis I receive amazing cards, letters, flowers and gifts from so many people: a beautiful note from my uni friend Jona in Southport, telling me he loves me dearly; texts from mums at the boys' primary school offering to help; a fabulous letter from the bloke who used to be in charge of the sports show I did on Channel 4 years ago, who now lives in California – I'm so happy to hear from him! A gorgeous letter from my old English teacher's husband, who I'd written to last year when Mrs Skinner, his dear wife, died of cancer; a tin of cakes from *Newsnight* and a note from their editor saying they were all 'rooting for me'; Facebook messages from my cousins, the Crossley family; a handwritten card from my other cousin, Mark Connor; a letter from one of my brother's close friends, and one from his mum too (her daughter, his sister, died of cancer, just a young woman); a friend we made through Oliver's football team, Steve, drops round with a card and good wishes; a long email arrives from Alison, one of my best friends at primary school, now living abroad, who's also had breast cancer, as had her mum – and so it goes on.

It's taken me having cancer to realise that 99.9 per cent of people are so very kind.

Plus a card arrives in the post from Sarah Corp, Rachel's sister, who has incurable cancer. It's realistic, selfless; she has an understanding that only those who have cancer can:

Dear Victoria

I'm so sorry to hear your news which I'm sure you're still digesting. I won't weigh in with wise advice as you'll already be getting plenty of that from all directions wanted and unwanted!! Besides, every type of this stupid disease is entirely different with different treatments and ailments. All I can offer is that you'll have good days and bad days; you'll panic and then other times feel like you're the only sane person in the room; you'll be handed more leaflets than you could ever want or attempt to read about something you never wanted to learn about; but you'll find a way of making sense of it all and getting on with it. In the meantime, just carry on enjoying the now, and your lovely family.

Lots of love,

Sarah Corp

Friday 28 August

With Mark, I go to see Mr Kothari, who hopefully is going to give us the results of the biopsy on the left side. I really look forward to these appointments for two reasons:

1. I respect him and enjoy talking to him
2. Seeing him means I get more information about the illness and therefore the treatment, and that means I'll be able to work out when it's all going to be over.

As usual, he shakes hands with Mark and me and welcomes us into his consultancy room. I check with him how his name is pronounced – is it a hard 't' in Kothari, or a 'th' as in 'the'? He says he really doesn't mind. I ask where he's from and when he came to Britain – Mumbai, in 1998. Sitting down and smiling, he asks how I am. And he really does want to know how I am, physically and mentally.

'Yes, I'm absolutely fine, thank you; I'm just impatient to know what the biopsy says.'

Mark has his pen ready to begin making notes in our 'cancer notebook'.

Mr Kothari begins. 'The biopsy shows that some cells in your left breast are atypical. They are not cancerous, they are not even precancerous, they are atypical.' There follows a conversation about the definition of 'atypical' – abnormal, unconventional, irregular – all negative-sounding words, but as Mr Kothari explains, most of us will have cells inside us that are atypical. It doesn't mean it's a bad thing, necessarily; it just means that because of my diagnosis, we're hyper-aware of anything that's even slightly unusual.

I raise the prospect of a double mastectomy, 'because it might help me psychologically'. By that I mean that if the left breast is also removed, perhaps the fear of breast cancer returning would be reduced, even eradicated?

'If you wish to have a double mastectomy, I will do that for you,' he says slowly and considerately. That takes me by surprise. Bloody hell, so it really is my choice. 'But it's also my job to point out to you that the left breast is healthy. The cells are not even precancerous. This is a breast with sensation, a real breast. Also, for simplicity, a single mastectomy followed by reconstruction using an implant is one of the most straightforward operations to perform, and to recover from.'

I ask him how long it takes to get back to normality after a mastectomy, compared to a double mastectomy – he thinks three weeks for the former, and six to eight for the latter.

We then have our first conversation about whether I will need chemotherapy and radiotherapy. He says he will only know when he's carried out the surgery and tested the lymph nodes under the right arm. Then he can make a recommendation, but at this stage, 'I'm thinking you might need more treatment, including taking a drug called tamoxifen which blocks oestrogen going to the breast.' My cancer is oestrogen-positive, so stopping this naturally occurring hormone reaching my cells and potentially turning them into cancer is a good thing.

Mark and I talk there and then about the pros and cons of a single mastectomy versus a double mastectomy. For such a vital decision, I feel as though this is a bit rushed, but we have to come to a conclusion before signing the consent form which gives permission for surgery to go ahead. What Mr Kothari says about the left side being 'a healthy breast' has an impact on me – why would you get rid of a part of your body that is OK, that has sensation, is real? And so within minutes I choose to have only the diseased breast removed, and sign the form. With my signature I'm agreeing that Mr Kothari scrapes the cancerous tissue out, preserves the skin and the nipple, tests to see definitively if cancer has spread to any lymph nodes and if it has, permission is given to remove the relevant ones – all while I'm under anaesthetic. I like the logical approach of doing as much as possible while knocked out.

After this formality is over, he says, 'So you've told the world you want to work through your treatment?'

I smile at him. 'Not quite . . . I've said I'll work as much as I can through treatment. You're not cross with me, are you, for informing "the world", as you put it?'

'No, no, not at all! Whatever helps you is the right thing for you, is absolutely perfect. I believe that whatever a patient needs to do to feel empowered is good for them and good for their recovery.'

The operation will either be 17 or 24 September. I'll receive a letter confirming when. I can't wait; I want the cancer out of me, and as we leave, I feel almost excited at the prospect of treatment beginning. The sooner it starts, the sooner it will be over.

Cathy, Paul and their boys, along with friends of theirs who've become friends of ours, John and Juliet and their son, come over in the evening. They are two families who definitely live life to the full. We all sit in the garden in the warmth, eating, drinking and chatting. These are the nights, with good friends who are a delight to be with, with whom we have such a laugh, that I am now savouring more than ever.

Saturday 29 August

Before we sit down at night to watch *House of Cards*, Mark tells me how lucky he feels to have us all – me, Lizzi, Joe, Oliver and Gracie, and how much he loves us.

Sunday 30 August

I go into work today to check my emails and get things in order for going back to work on Tuesday. There are so many wonderfully kind emails from colleagues I know and don't know from around the BBC, and from our viewers, that I spend the next two hours replying to as many as I can. They don't half give me a lift.

Tuesday 1 September

By coincidence, I'd booked off the last three weeks of work as leave months and months ago, never for a moment thinking I'd be spending some of it inside hospitals being tested to see how much cancer there is in me. Today it's officially back to work. I wonder if people will feel they can mention cancer to me, or will choose to say nothing to avoid any awkwardness? I'll be happy if colleagues ask how I am; it's exactly what I'd do if the roles were reversed. When I get to New Broadcasting House at 5 a.m., it feels so good to be back. Lovely to see the team, and they're really delighted to see me. Our director Barry gives me a great big hug too. The programme itself has some strong content, and I thank viewers on air for their many wonderful and supportive messages.

Later on at home, Outra rings – my operation is 24 September. Yes. I'm relieved finally to have a date. I get my diary out, see what day of the week it will be, and text Louisa to let her know I won't be able to present our programme from that date for – three weeks? Four weeks? It depends how long I take to heal, I suppose. Even though I hate the thought of being out cold under the anaesthetic (I worry about not waking up), I can't wait for this surgery. As Cathy said back in the summer, 'Just get the fecker out!'

Wednesday 2 September

I love Mark.

Thursday 3 September

Oliver's first day at secondary school. Considering he is dealing with me having a cancer diagnosis, as well as apprehension about starting a new school, he is buoyant. We are bringing up a resilient boy, and I'm very proud of that.

After today's programme, Louisa and I have a coffee sitting outside Caffè Nero next door to the BBC. Our boss, James Harding, joins us unexpectedly. He asks lots of questions about the treatment and diagnosis, and then says his 'heart leapt' when he saw me back on TV yesterday, and that he thinks I'm 'handling this whole thing brilliantly'. It's a very generous thing to say, and I thank him for his incredible support.

I pick up Joe from school at 3.05 p.m., and Ollie from the train station at 4.30 p.m., eager to see how his first day has gone. As he walks towards the car, well turned out in his brand-new uniform and tall for his age, he seems far more mature than his eleven years. Mark says he looks like he's going to a business meeting. He tells us he enjoyed the day and describes his teachers as 'enthusiastic', which I'm really pleased to hear.

Friday 4 September

Mark's done everything this week: shopping, cooking, the washing, running the boys to school/train station in the morning, as well as going to work. I feel guilty, and resolve to do more.

Saturday 5 September

We all watch *Strictly* with an Indian takeaway and Gracie curled up next to us on the sofa. Such simple things give me so much pleasure.

Sunday 6 September

Nick comes over from Wiltshire and brings my mum too, who's been staying with him. We talk on the phone most days, but this is the first time I've seen them since being diagnosed. Both give me the biggest hugs ever, and I think they're mildly surprised to see how well I'm looking. Obviously there's a significant 'so how are you?' (me: 'really fine, actually, completely fine'), and we talk about the forthcoming operation, but apart from that we barely mention cancer, which is very refreshing.

Monday 14 September

On our programme today we broadcast a beautiful film we've made, featuring twin brothers who'd been separated as babies in Germany during the Second World War, reuniting for the first time after seventy years. Seventy years! Our cameras were there to capture the moment, along with our reporter Dan Johnson and producer Jonathan Josephs. It's one of the most moving stories I've ever come across.

Wednesday 16 September

A young woman who had her leg amputated after being on the Alton Towers ride that crashed gives her first-ever interview to us today. She's called Vicky Balch, and she's understated and composed as she tells our audience what happened when the carriage she was riding in hit an empty one that had got stuck on the tracks ahead. She describes the horrific, searing pain on impact; the fact that it took four hours to get her out; her belief that while she was being rescued she thought she 'wasn't going to make it'; and about the amputation she was forced to have after getting an infection. She tells me that when she looked down after coming round from the anaesthetic, 'it was a relief; it was a relief not to have it there . . . because eventually I'd be able to walk again with a prosthetic leg'. And she *is* now walking, using an artificial limb and crutches.

Her interview prompts a huge reaction from our audience – emails and tweets and WhatsApp messages pour in, expressing their admiration for this rational, determined young woman. Our interview ran on the 6 p.m. and 10 p.m. BBC news too.

The NHS saved this woman's life. In very different circumstances, it occurs to me that the NHS is saving mine too.

Friday 18 September

Our 'twins reunited' film has now been shared on Facebook nearly ten million times. Wow.

Saturday 19 September

On the way back from dropping Ollie off at a friend's party, I begin to cry in the car. My operation is next week, and I suddenly feel as though I can't cope with it. It's the first time since I received the diagnosis that the words 'I can't do this' come into my head. I'm frightened of not waking up from the anaesthetic, of never seeing my family again, and I want to pause everything so that time stands still and next Thursday doesn't arrive. When I get home Mark gives me a hug and tells me in a kindly voice, 'I'm really sorry, darlin', but we want you to stay alive, and this operation will enable you to do that.' He's right, of course; I know that. But I can't do it.

To stop myself from being overwhelmed by these thoughts, I actually have to prohibit my mind visualising me lying on an operating table, anaesthetised, undergoing surgery. I simply block it out while keeping myself busy and distracted – reading, watching TV, painting my nails and walking Gracie.

Sunday 20 September

We watch Ollie play football for his local club, Halliford Colts, and he scores five goals in a 6–3 thriller. There aren't many feelings that match seeing your son score a beautiful goal in a game of football. Mark and I are so pleased for him; it's gratifying to see his confidence soar.

Unusually I'm exhausted in the afternoon, way, way more than I should be, given I've done very little all weekend. It must be the cancer.

I can't believe I've got cancer.

Monday 21 September

I am definitely experiencing pre-op nerves, or something. While I'm in the office trying to prepare for today's programme by reading various briefs, doubts force their way into my head about whether I should have an implant at all. Why would I want something foreign inside me? What if that goes wrong? I can't work out if I really mean it, or if it's just fear of what's to come forcing me to distance myself from reality and pretend it's not happening.

If I don't have an implant I could simply be flat on one side, with no nipple and a smile-shaped scar. I could live with that.

Tuesday 22 September

It's my last programme for a few weeks, and it's a good one because one of our top reporters, Jim Reed, has an exclusive story about the RSPCA: MPs are going to examine whether the charity should be able to continue both investigating and prosecuting cases of animal cruelty. Separately, the Director of Public Prosecutions, Alison Saunders, appears on the programme too today, talking about sexual consent ahead of Freshers' Week at universities up and down the country. I put this scenario to her: two people are really drunk, they're not unconscious, both think the other consented to sex, and in the morning the woman wakes up, has no recollection of consenting and thinks she might have been raped. I ask if this would lead to a man being prosecuted for rape. Ms Saunders says she thinks that if she were the woman, she might go to a support group, ask for some help and talk it through with someone.

That'll be in tomorrow's papers.

Walking out the door of the BBC, I contemplate the time off in front of me that isn't for a holiday or a family occasion, but for cancer treatment. Louisa takes me to the Langham Hotel across the road for a glass of champagne before we meet our friend from Radio 5 Live, Jonny Crawford, at The Ivy. It's a kind of pre-op blowout (any excuse), and we have a magnificent time gossiping, laughing and occasionally expressing disbelief that I've got cancer. The friendship of decent people makes me feel very secure.

Before bed, I talk through with Mark one last time whether I should have the implant on Thursday. I reach the conclusion that, as I trust the safety and efficacy of them, I may as well get everything done in one go. It really was nerves making me have doubts.

Wednesday 23 September

I don't stop today. Who knew there was so much to get organised before a mastectomy? Included on my list of jobs for the day are: going to the hospital to have radioactive material inserted into my nipple (sounds horrific, but turns out not to be) which will help show up definitively which, if any, lymph nodes are cancerous while I'm being operated on. I drive to Ashford Hospital and ask at reception where I need to go for the appointment. She tells me it's at the other hospital site, at St Peter's, a twenty-minute drive away. I'm now going to be late, and I'm harassed. The only way I can keep calm on the drive is to turn the radio off and hide the clock on the dashboard so I can't actually hear or see what time it is. If I miss this appointment I can't have the operation tomorrow, and more than anything in the world I want to get it over with.

By the time I arrive there's a message on my mobile from the nurse (born in Glasgow, she tells me later) reminding me that I have a 2 p.m. appointment. It's a relief to get there, get into the room, whip my top off and start the process of blue dye being injected into my right breast, the one that's being removed tomorrow. After a needleful of anaesthetic, the dye-injecting bit isn't painful, and once it's in I have to spend the next thirty minutes or so massaging my skin so the ink spreads around inside. Great – I'm going to be late picking Joe up from school now.

I send my boss Keith a text saying that if anything goes wrong tomorrow, please can he find out if Mark, as my partner, and the children, are entitled to any kind of death-in-service payment. He rings immediately and says, 'Nothing is going to go wrong, but if it helps put your mind at rest, then of course I'll find out.' He's a legend.

My sister Alex is at mine when I get home; she's going to look after the boys in the morning and drop them at school and at the station, as we have to leave early for the hospital.

I'm poor company in the evening, tense and snappy. It's be-cause I'm afraid – not about the operation itself, I have no doubt that Mr Kothari will scrape every last cancerous cell out of me – but about being anaesthetised and something going wrong so that I never wake up. I know my friend Hayley was right when she patiently pointed out to me the other week that millions of people wake up from having operations every single day. But still, I'm grimly anxious about it.

Good luck flowers arrive from Paul, Cathy, John, Juliet and all their boys.

Before sleeping, I write a letter each to my boys. I want them to know how much I love them. I tell Mark these will be in my bedside drawer, and he's to give them to Oliver and Joe should anything happen to me. He tells me nothing bad is going to happen, but still manages to humour me because he knows it's something I need to do. It's surreal and distressing putting into words how special they are, thinking they will read this if I don't wake up after surgery. I'm irritated with myself because I know what I'm doing is absurd, but this final task before bed makes sense to me right this second. I'm doing this 'just in case', not because I think it really will happen.

To Oliver, I write that, as our firstborn son, he changed the lives of Mark and me completely. Holding him in my arms, I could not believe it was possible to love another human being as much as I loved him. I ask him to take my determination forward in his own life; tell him to love life, love the people around him, his wonderful brother, his amazing sis, his magnificent dad. And his cousins, aunties, uncles, godparents and our super-special family friends.

To Joe, I write about his speedy arrival on 5 December 2006; me getting to the delivery room at 3.15 p.m. and his being born just ten minutes later at 3.25 p.m. (he never tires of hearing about it), and about how he completed our family. I remind him what a compassionate, warm-hearted, sensitive, clever boy he is, and how he's always to keep that kindness, because it makes other people feel very special.

I silently weep as I seal both letters in envelopes and put them in my bedside drawer. Now I can sleep.

Thursday 24 September

As soon as I wake I'm on edge. I can barely speak. We get dressed, and say our goodbyes to Alex and the boys. It isn't over the top or emotional; just 'love you, see you this afternoon when you finish school', and I thank Alex for taking care of them. I read the messages on my phone from friends and family wishing me luck. It reminds me that they're anxious too.

Mark and I arrive at Ashford Hospital at 7.30 a.m. sharp and are shown into a cramped, ugly waiting room. Illuminated with harsh strip lighting, cold, an American quiz show blaring out of the huge TV and a hospital trolley taking up a lot of space in the corner, everything feels jarring and uncomfortable. It's not exactly the right environment to prepare for a four-hour oper-ation. But then, what is right? I look around at my fellow patients and try to work out if they are all waiting for mastectomies. No one seems particularly nervous; most are drawn to the noise of the telly.

After about forty-five minutes or so, an anaesthetist calls my name and Mark and I are taken next door. He introduces himself

– he's called Mark, too, and his accent is Australian, although he's lived here for years. He goes through my personal details and then explains what he is going to do today, what his role is, what will happen to me and asks if I understand and am OK with it all. I am, yes, and all I want to know in return is what time I will be going down to theatre. He doesn't know exactly, but thinks it might be around midday, as Mr Kothari has one or two minor ops to do first. Another four hours or so to wait – it's too long; I need it to begin. He tells me he's really enjoyed listening to me on Radio 5 Live over the years. That breaks the tension a little, and I smile for the first time today and thank him.

We're sent back to the horrible waiting room, and I can't bear the quiz show noise so ask my fellow patients and their relatives if they'd mind if I put BBC *Breakfast* on, please. They're all fine with that.

After another quarter of an hour or so, a man who introduces himself as a senior house officer calls us over to the edge of the room, and as we perch on the hospital trolley he carefully checks my name, date of birth and address. I'm not sure why; we've already done this. I ask where he's from: Thailand. We sit down again and I ask those left in the waiting room if they'd mind if I changed the channel to BBC2 (because our programme will be starting soon). Before it does, Mr Kothari walks in with a big smile on his face, formally greets us and all the tension within me seems to dissipate. He ushers us into a tiny office with a desk, two chairs and shelves full of files and boxes and explains that they're short of rooms, so he's 'having to improvise'. There are too many people in a very small space – Mark, me, Mr Kothari, a registrar, a nurse and Outra, who, although she's smiling, also seems a little tense. I'm always happy to see her and find her presence reassuring. Matter-of-factly I remove my silk shirt and bra, and Mr Kothari gets a black felt tip from his inside pocket and draws the line under my right breast where he will make the incision with his knife later. Then on my right arm he draws an arrow pointing upward – ie, this is the side we are operating on. I admire the simplicity of this preparation. We have a final chat, and he explains that I'm second on the list for surgery, so it won't be long now – maybe an hour, an hour and a half away. Before everyone leaves, I ask if I can take a photo of the team as a record of who's treating me. It's the journalist in me documenting one of the most significant occasions in my own life. Mark jokes that I never stop working.

Outra, as our breast cancer nurse, stays with us and we take the opportunity to ask her about her life, her partner, her background, what she wants to do in the future and why she loves her job. Outra's from Trinidad; she's almost fifty but looks ten years younger and has been with Mitch for twenty-seven years. Together they both want to retire eventually to Panama. She is one of the warmest people we've ever met. After twenty-five minutes or so, another member of staff arrives and leads us, not back to the waiting room, but to a separate small room with a bed, sink and large window. This is where I will be for the next twenty-four hours, and I'm so relieved; it's just Mark and me, on our own, with space to collect our thoughts.

A nurse called Surjit (from India) bustles in and sits down, ready to go through the four- or five-page admissions form with me. Questions range from my date of birth to whether I'm al-lergic to anything to whether I could be pregnant. She diligently ticks off each answer. Every now and again Mark says something vaguely witty in answer to her question, which makes me laugh, but Surjit is taking her job far too seriously to do much smiling. I change into one of those white hospital gowns with minute blue diamond shapes all over it that opens at the back, and put on some paper pants and some bluey-green surgical stockings, which go from my ankles to my knees (to stop clotting while I'm lying flat on my back for hours undergoing surgery). The stockings are then wrapped in white cricket-type pads with Velcro straps. She attaches a cannula to the top of my left hand. Mark and I joke about the unattractive garments I'm being forced to wear, but he says it makes him love me even more.

I don't feel tense any more. I can't wait for this to happen. This is going to get rid of my cancer. When I wake up I will have completed the main treatment for eradicating this disease. I actually feel excited, with a bit of apprehension thrown in. Maybe it's the adrenaline.

At 10.30 a.m. Brenda (England) and Surjit both wheel me down on my hospital bed to theatre. I feel slightly embarrassed and say, 'I don't feel ill, you know; I can walk if it helps.' They explain that this is the bed they will bring me back to the room on, after surgery, so they need me on it now. Mark is alongside me, telling me he'll be here when I wake up. In two minutes we are outside the plastic double doors which lead to the anaesthetists' room.

'I love you,' Mark says.

'I love you,' I reply.

We kiss, and Mark tells me to be strong. I have tears in my eyes, because this feels like a big deal.

As the bed is pushed through the doors, I twist round to get a final look at Mark and we blow each other kisses and smile. Australian anaesthetist Mark introduces me to his colleague,

Linda. They verify my name and date of birth and explain that soon the room will start spinning. I say, 'Yep, I can see everything spinning now.' And then I'm out.

'Victoria! Victoria, can you hear me? Victoria!'

I'm aware of a voice miles away calling my name, and as I begin to stir, I realise it's a nurse standing right next to me. Why is she trying to wake me up when I'm so knackered? After a minute or so, I open my eyes gradually and start to focus. I can see a clock on the wall in front of me: a quarter to three – Joe will be finishing school soon. Then I realise – shit, it's done, the op is over. Wow. I feel like I've been under for two minutes, not four hours. Huge relief envelops me, and I lie there feeling intensely grateful and some tears run down my face. Pretty much straight away I'm wheeled back to the room where Mark is waiting. As soon as I see him my heart leaps – he comes over to the bed, hugs me and is smiling so broadly it's infectious. We've done it. And I woke up. And the cancer's gone. It's amazing to see him, amazing that it's over. I can't believe it. I feel liberated.

Pain – there is some pain on the right side of my chest – like someone's punched me there and I can't lean on that side, but that is it. Mostly I feel good, and I'm full of chat – I just cannot stop talking. About how it's over, about how quick it was, about the children and what time they're getting here, about how I feel and about how much I love Mark. Happily patient, he indulges my ramblings. We both look together at my bandaged chest, discoloured by the blue dye that was injected into me yesterday. Obviously we can't see what my skin, or what the implant, looks like. I ask how the last few hours have been for him, and he says it's been hard. He's felt incredibly anxious the whole time;

he's been texting my mum and brother, sister and friends to let them know when the op started and then again as soon as he heard I'd woken up. But yep, it was bloody hard wondering if I was going to be OK. I thank him for taking care of me, and for everything.

After an hour or so, Mark goes to get the boys, who've been picked up from school by Ben. I ring my mum, and she is so delighted to hear my voice she starts to cry down the phone. Then I text my friends, and Nick and Alex, and get gorgeous messages back from them, and I text my bosses and the people on our programme team.

Constantly, nurses are popping in to see if I need help going to the loo (the anaesthetic means I can't stand up by myself), to ask what I would like for tea and do I need more painkillers. Outra comes to check on me and we have a chat – she is all smiles as usual. Then Mr Kothari comes to visit, still dressed in his green surgical cap and gown.

'Thank you so, so much, I am so grateful to you,' I tell him emotionally, before asking how it went.

'Perfect,' he announces, adding that as well as the cancerous tissue in the breast he removed, he also took out three lymph nodes under my arm to analyse them and see if any cancer cells were present. (Many types of cancer spread through the lymph nodes – the lymph node closest to the cancer is called the sentinel node; taking it out is called a sentinel lymph node biopsy.)

He explains that there were microscopic cancer cells attached to two out of the three nodes. However, because they were so tiny, that suggested it was unnecessary to remove any more nodes from my armpit while I was under the anaesthetic, because expertise gained over decades means it's unlikely other nodes would be affected (and removing nodes when you don't need to can lead to something called lymphoedema in the arm – painful swelling, effectively).

Suddenly my mood darkens.

'So the cancer has spread?' I shoot back rapidly with fear in my voice.

'No, it has not spread. Let me explain again.'

He draws me a quick sketch showing the breast in relation to the lymph nodes, and which nodes he took out. The three he removed form a gateway to the rest of the lymph nodes – which he draws to resemble a bunch of grapes.

For some reason I'm missing the point, as well as struggling to keep calm, and ask rather curtly, 'Well, how do you know it was only on two of them; how do you know the cancerous stuff hasn't attached to more lymph nodes?'

'Because of the *three* we removed to test; tiny, tiny cancerous cells were on only *two* of them, and not on the third, which is in exactly the same area. Research evidence gained from years of experience suggests that if the sentinel lymph node biopsy shows the nodes are touched by only tiny amounts of cancer, it's unlikely to have spread to others. Therefore removing more lymph nodes is considered unnecessary in contemporary prac- tice. And the bottom line is, they've now gone, *and* the tumour's gone.'

I'm reassured. I think.

The next thing I want to know is who was in theatre work- ing on me. Mr Kothari runs through the rest of his team: the registrar Richard (England), the senior house officer Aphiwat (Thailand), two scrub nurses, Cherry (the Philippines) and Anita

(India), Mark the Australian anaesthetist and Linda the English anaesthetist, plus team leader Alice (also from India). So many people drawn from all over the world who are helping me get better. I'm in awe of them.

Finally my boys arrive with Ben and Mark. My two delicious, divine little boys who, last night, I was writing love letters to in case I never woke up from surgery. My anxieties seem so absurd now they're here, vivid and warm, in front of me. We hug for ages. They hand over various gifts: a plant, sushi, crisps, water and a 'get well' card. Although they are asking lots of questions – how are you? does it hurt? what are those plastic things coming out of you? – they are both subdued. They are never, ever subdued. What they are seeing for the first time in their lives is me in weird hospital garb, in a high, uncomfortable-looking bed, unable to move and with two plastic tubes collecting blood protruding from my right breast, which is covered in bandages. It's probably making them feel unsure, insecure and anxious, and I do everything I can to gently rub out those fears by being upbeat and smiley and telling them that it's all gone very well and that I'll be back home tomorrow. I ask how school was, and Joe explains he got 'a bit emotional, and his teacher had been kind to him'. So I cuddle him some more. Ben asks questions too, and expresses surprise at how awake and talkative I am, how apparently normal I'm being. He compares me with Natalie after her surgery a few years ago and says that already I'm doing really well. As time passes, Oliver becomes his normal self again – bold and chatty, which is a relief.

They all stay for about an hour and half, and suddenly, at around seven o'clock, my body feels fatigued. We say our good-byes, but Joe is upset because he doesn't want to leave me there;

he wants me to come home with them now. As he walks out of the door he keeps turning round and stretching out his hand towards me, pleading with me to come.

'Darling, I can't, but I'll be back tomorrow, and when you get home from school I will be there waiting for you.' Even after they've all walked up the corridor, Joe runs back to give me one last hug with tears in his eyes.

'I love you,' he says, his face buried in the good side of my chest. I can feel my hospital gown getting damp from his tears.

'I love you more,' I tell him, breathing in the smell of his hair. He hangs onto me like a tired boxer hangs onto his opponent in the tenth round, until I gently encourage him to follow his dad and brother, promising that they'll look after him and that tomorrow we'll be back together again as a family in our home.

Then there is quiet. In the room and in my head. I lie there thinking 'shit, I've just had a mastectomy and physically I feel . . . all right'.

But it's more than 'all right'. Mentally I'm on a high.

I open the boys' get well cards, and Oliver's makes me smile in particular:

To Mummy

I bl***y love you. Please get better soon and still live life in the same way.

Love, Oliver

He knows he shouldn't use that word; he also knows he can get away with it in the context of saying 'I love you' when I've just come round from a four-hour op! I place them on my bedside table so they'll be the last thing I see when I go to sleep and the first thing I see when I wake up tomorrow.

I ring Louisa, and she is so happy to hear from me. I talk her through the day, and how I'm feeling now, and she says she can't believe how energetic I sound. God, I love adrenaline. I call Nick and Alex, then ring Mark to check he's OK and the boys are OK. Everyone catches my mood and is upbeat, and I love it.

At about eight-ish, I start thinking about filming something and recording a few thoughts about how I'm feeling. It's the first step to trying to do what I considered doing weeks ago – demystifying this, if that's possible. Before today, I had little idea of what a mastectomy actually involves – now I can share some of my experience. I want to be factual, honest and open, and most importantly, acknowledge that this is my own personal experience. Everyone is different, and depending on their diagnosis, will approach it in a variety of ways.

I'd come prepared to do this, and I begin by writing two signs in black felt tip on some drawing paper that Mark got me from the Tesco opposite the hospital. The first one reads, 'This morning I had breast cancer'. The second one reads, 'This evening I don't'. I film myself holding them up to the three-by-three-inch GoPro camera. Then I think about the words I am going to say. I'll feel really stupid if a nurse walks in right now and sees me talking to myself, so I get on with it.

7.55 p.m.: 'I'm in hospital, as you can see. I'm in a hospital room, and today I had a mastectomy, and . . . I feel . . . all right. I can't believe it. I went under the anaesthetic at about a quarter to eleven this morning, and woke up at about a quarter to three, cos I remember looking at the clock and thinking, oh, the children will be coming out of school soon . . . and . . . um . . . I feel all right, I can't believe it. The NHS staff have been awesome; they are so inspiring, and so caring, and I feel so grateful to them.

'When I woke up from the anaesthetic I did cry because it was just a relief, *such* a relief. The malignant tumour in my right breast has gone. And two or three lymph nodes have gone. I, er, feel a bit groggy from the anaesthetic, but that's obviously completely normal . . . and my two boys have been here, and my partner and a friend of ours, Ben, and it was amazing to see them, and, yeah [big sigh] . . . I can't believe it, really.'

I'm aware I'm speaking quite slowly as I think about what I'm saying, because I'm not as alert as normal. I sigh with relief a lot, too, because I kind of can't believe that a surgeon has performed a life-saving operation on me and here I am, absolutely fine, several hours later.

'The word "cancer" has such a chilling effect on people, me included, but I've learned over the last few weeks that this illness does not have to be elevated to some uber-powerful status. It's simply an illness which the NHS treats with expertise and care.'

I go on to say that for me, and it is only my personal experience, having a mastectomy is totally doable, and describe how they inserted the implant:

'They cut underneath the breast, then they draw all the cancer out, scrape it out, cut it out, whatever, and then underneath the skin they put the implant and then draw the skin, they pull the skin over the implant . . . and right at the bottom is a sort of sling, or mesh sling, and my skin, if all goes well, will merge with the mesh and will hopefully look reasonably natural. I mean, yeah, that's . . . amazing, isn't it? That. Is. Amazing.'

Then I have a break and lie there peacefully.

Half an hour or so later, I film the side of my right breast, showing the dressings and the blue dye which has left my skin looking bruised and discoloured, plus the plaster under my arm where an incision has been made to remove those lymph nodes. I film the drains, too, which are filled with my blood. As I reach down the side of the bed to pull the plastic pouch up into which the fluid is draining, a pain shoots up my right side. Trying to stretch down isn't the brightest idea.

This filming thing is giving me a purpose, but now I need to get some sleep if I can. I can't. I pull the cord which alerts the staff that I need a bit of help getting to the loo, and have a good chat with the staff nurse, who's from St Helen's; she's jolly, no-nonsense and I like her attitude.

Around 11 p.m. I'm in the mood for chatting, so phone Louisa again, thinking she'll be the only one awake at this time. She's out with the Radio 1 *Newsbeat* crowd, and it sounds noisy and fun where they are. She says she can't believe I'm still awake, sounding lively and alert, so we try to work out why. It's partly because of the noise of the pumps working the 'cricket pads' to keep massaging my legs so they don't get clots. But mostly I'm buzzing because the op is over.

Friday 25 September

By midnight I'm really tired and also starving, so I eat some of the sushi the boys brought me earlier. Finally, at about 1 a.m., I fall asleep.

It doesn't last long, and around 3.30 a.m. I'm awake. Wide

awake. I want to get on with things, start packing and go home. I go to the loo, on my own this time so very slowly, clean my teeth and put some lipstick on. It always makes me feel good, putting on my lippy. Before every radio programme I ever presented I'd always redo my lipstick a minute before going on air. I write my diary and then I film a bit more.

'The kind of drugs I've been given to help with the pain are ibuprofen, paracetamol and a tiny little bit of morphine. The pain reminds me of – if you've got boys this is bound to have happened to you – when, if you're playing football with your boys and they tackle you a little bit too hard and they run into you and bash you because they don't realise that your chest is so sensitive – it's that kind of pain, which is just achy and dull but not searing, not by any stretch of the imagination.'

Then more sleep. Finally it's the morning, and I can crack on with the day. I ring Mark and the boys, my mum, and text everyone else. A nurse comes in with more painkillers and asks what I'd like for breakfast. While I'm waiting, I do a bit more filming to explain how I'm feeling the morning after surgery – almost pain-free, as it happens, because of the drugs. My right arm is immobile and useless, and I'm very happy to be going home.

At about half nine, Mr Kothari and Outra return to check on me, and it's lovely to see them.

'I feel absolutely great, honestly.'

'What about the pain?'

'Totally fine; yes, it's there, but it's not much, considering.'

Then Mr Kothari talks about the possibility of chemotherapy and radiotherapy. He thinks it will be likely I'll have both, but we need to wait for the pathology report, which will give us for the first time detailed, accurate information about the cancerous tissue that was removed from me. Right now I'm sanguine about the prospect of both, because if it helps reduce the chances of this cancer returning, then it's got to be done.

Outra stays longer in order to explain how the drains work and what I need to do to empty them each morning. For about a minute it feels complicated, but it isn't. At the bottom of each tube is a largish plastic peg, which I close to pinch the tube together to stop it leaking or open to let the fluid run down it into the plastic ball attached to the bottom of the tube. I am to close the peg before squeezing the contents of the ball into a measuring jug; I record how much fluid there is before undoing the clip to allow the fluid to flow freely down the tube into the plastic ball again. And I do that at the same time each morning. The idea is to check that the fluid is reducing each day, before eventually removing the drains altogether. As Outra changes my dressings, I thank her profusely; I think I love her, actually. She says, 'You've done really well,' and I have tears in my eyes.

Mark arrives at about eleven-ish, with masses of glorious fruit in a huge basket which we give to the staff on the ward. He'd asked one of the nurses yesterday what would be a suitable gift and she said no chocolates, please – they have an office full of chocolates donated by patients. I adore his thoughtfulness.

On the drive home, as familiar roads pass in a blur, I hold Mark's hand and we beam at each other and say, 'We've done it.' We feel utterly triumphant.

I crash out on the sofa and the next thing I know, Joe, all smiley and delighted, is alongside me desperate to give me a hug – but he knows to hug the left side, and he does it very tenderly. Then

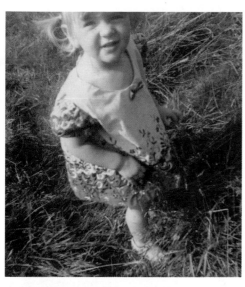

Me, aged two, growing up in Lancashire.

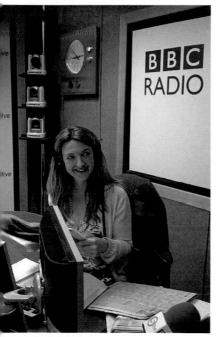

I worked at BBC Radio 5 Live for 16 years and loved it – particularly the 5 Live listeners.

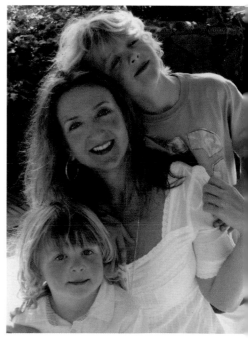

Me and our two golden* boys, Joe and Oliver (*they're not always golden!).

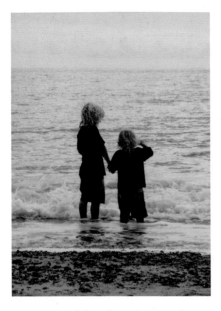

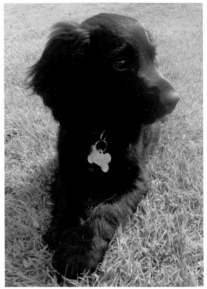

Not so much brothers-in-arms but brothers at sea.

Graceful Gracie – a beautiful puppy.

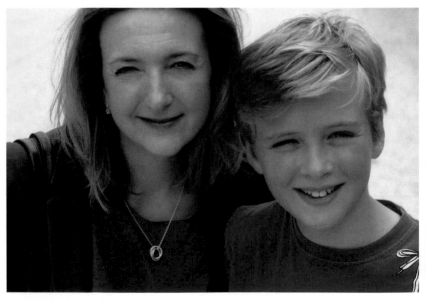

At Cliveden. Is it obvious I'm wondering how many more days out with my family I would get like this?

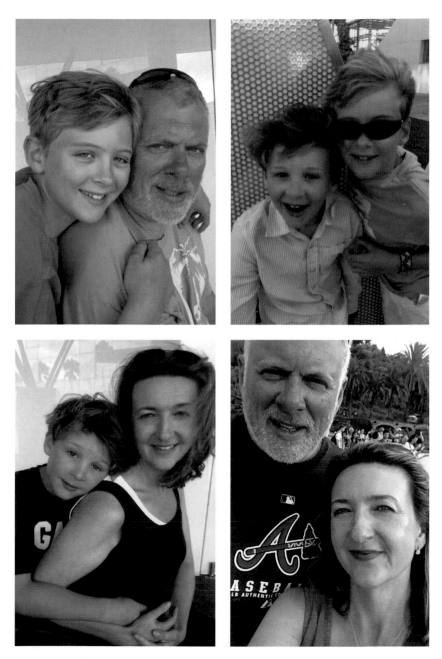

Barcelona: the holiday just after my diagnosis. I had a brilliant time with the three most important people in my life.

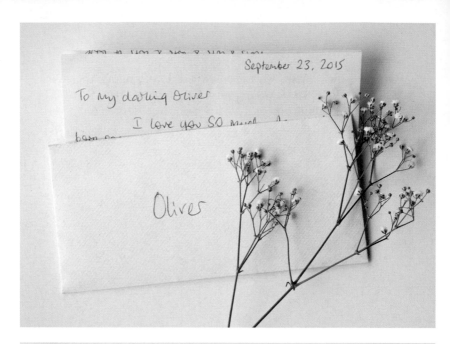

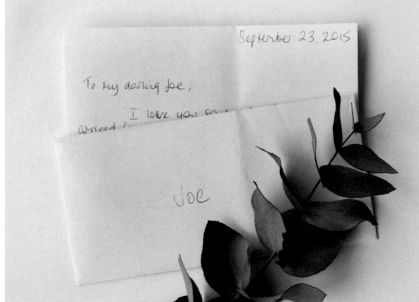

Letters to my children written the night before surgery; letters I hoped they would never have to read.

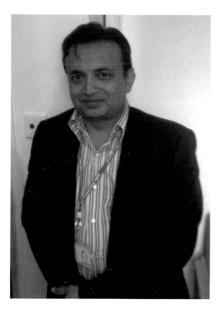

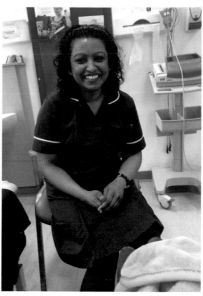

The surgeon who saved my life, Manish Kothari.

Outra – a nursing legend. I love her.

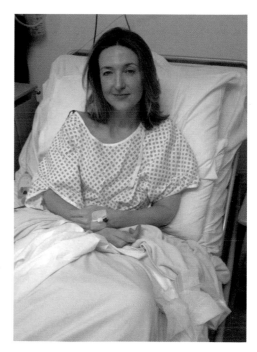

An hour before surgery. I look nervous but couldn't wait to 'get the fecker out', as my friend Cathy put it.

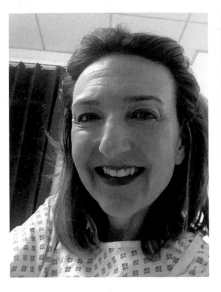

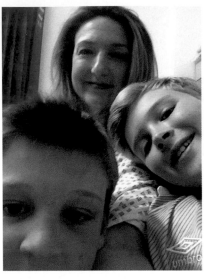

Happy 1: Hours after surgery I put some lipstick on and sent this pic to all my family and friends.

Happy 2: They think it's all over – but chemo is still to come.

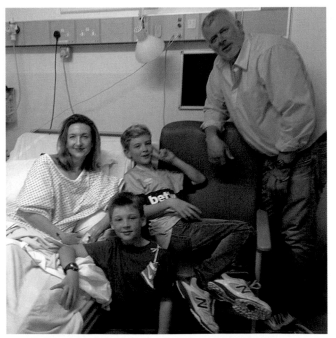

Happy 3: Me, Mark, Oliver and Joe – one relieved family.

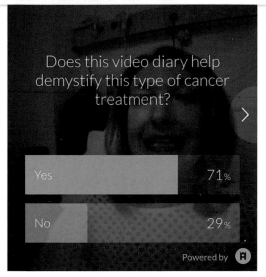

Does this video diary help demystify this type of cancer treatment?

Yes 71%

No 29%

Powered by

Not quite a landslide, but I'm happy with the result.

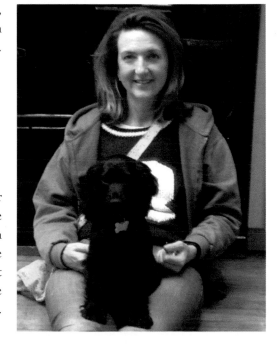

Right A few days after surgery sitting on the kitchen floor with Gracie; she made me feel calm thoughout treatment (note the drains bag).

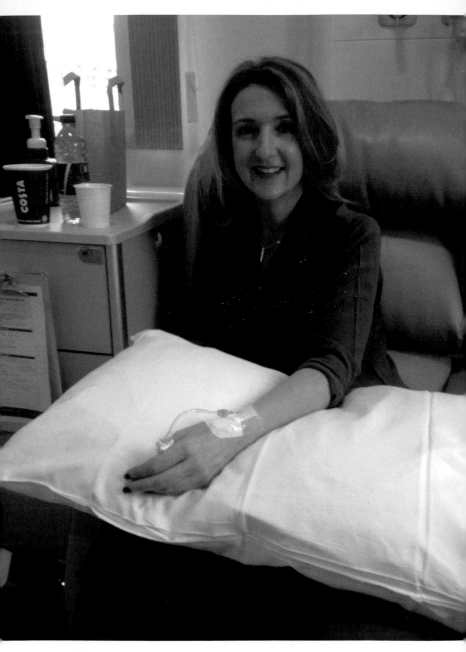

Just before my first chemo session – when I look at this photo I still miss my hair.

he looks around cautiously and whispers, inquisitively, 'Are there some nurses here?'

'Yes, and they're all hiding in your bedroom.' He grins.

When Ollie arrives back from school, he too is over the moon to have me home. To him it represents everything being back to normal. He gently hugs me on one side. It's good to be back with my family.

Saturday 26 September

I slept a little last night, but it's quite tricky sleeping on your back. The hardest thing is getting out of bed – any of the usual, swift movements aren't possible because even a tiny pull in the wrong direction hurts my chest, and you've got to collect up the pair of drains, too, and carry those around with you like some bizarre bodily appendage. So it's the left leg out onto the floor first, then I slowly pull myself up before trying to swing my right leg round and off the bed. Dressing takes some time, but once I am dressed, I sling a brown leather bag diagonally across me and place the plastic balls attached to the drains inside. I'm grateful to Jill for that tip, and to a kind woman on twitter (@draindollies), who sent me two pretty handmade bags I'll use, depending on what I'm wearing.

There's a West Ham home game today, and Mark would normally take our boys and meet up with all the other dads and their children, but today Paul is taking our two, because Ben, having nursed Natalie after her lumpectomy several years ago, is emphatic. 'No, mate, you're gonna have to miss that one, because you'll need to be around to look after Victoria.' I was really happy for Mark to go to the football, but as it happens I couldn't have walked Gracie in case she pulled me as I held her lead. Other things I can't do: drive, pick up a thick book, a laptop or hold the shower head to wash my hair. The most comfortable and comforting way to move around is by holding my right arm close to my body as though it's in a sling (which it isn't). It's taking time to get used to this.

Sunday 27 September

It's two months and a day since my breast collapsed. It's now no longer there, and I don't miss it one bit.

Paul and Cathy come round, and I fill them in on the op and how I'm feeling: chipper.

Monday 28 September

The mornings are quite slow – it takes a while to get up and bathed and dressed because everything I do has to be done carefully to avoid causing pain or discomfort. I wear a shirt because it's easier to get on and off compared to a top that you have to push your arms through. Then I 'do the drains' – empty and measure the fluid, which takes about a quarter of an hour, and record it in my 'drain logbook'. In the last 24 hours, I've emptied 26 ml from one drain and 17 ml from the other. Is this good? Not good enough? Who knows?

Flowers arrive from Keith at work – 'We miss you', he writes. Flowers arrive from the parents of children in Joe's class at school. Everyone's thoughtfulness is overwhelming.

My longest-standing friend, Helena, visits with Lola, her cockapoo. Helena and I met at Liverpool University in 1986 and have been friends ever since. Gracie tries to engage Lola in a game of chase around the garden, but Lola's been there, done that and isn't bothered. Helena talks to me about wigs – it's the first conversation I've had, really, with anyone about potentially losing my hair and how I'll cope with that in practical terms. Having no idea of what's to come, I'm blasé about getting one. She suggests a place in Richmond that her friend went to, called Amiwigs. 'Speak to the boss, Amy Holt, and tell her she's been recommended by Francesca. Francesca said she was absolutely brilliant.' I talk breezily about making an appointment sometime soonish. We laugh childishly about the prospect of me wearing a wig. Later, Juliet arrives with cake.

Tuesday 29 September

It's a beautiful, warm, autumnal day and outside, as Gracie rolls around in the leaves, I record the final bit of my first video diary.

'It's five days since I've had the mastectomy, and Gracie and I are messing about. There's not that much pain, to be honest, five days on. There's the odd twinge, or if you pull yourself really sharply – I tried to get out of the way of stepping on Gracie by accident, and it pulled on my right side. I'm restricted in my movement, but I'm up and about, I can walk and I can do all that sort of stuff, but I can't really use my right-hand side . . . so that's slightly frustrating, but not the end of the world.'

I go on to talk about what's to come in a few weeks – analysis of the cancerous tissue that was inside, that will tell me whether I need chemotherapy and/or radiotherapy, which I'm not nervous or fearful about because it's simply the next stage of the process.

It occurs to me that I haven't actually felt ill, not once, yet, which is bizarre considering how drastic removing a breast actually is. All in all, I'm feeling positive because there's no reason not to feel positive.

I switch off the camera, but then press record again almost immediately.

'I've just put the camera back on because the one thing that I haven't said, which is my overriding emotion, is that I have to make sure this cancer doesn't come back.'

I feel strongly about this – at the moment, this is my new focus in life.

We spend the evening after the children have gone to bed watching *House of Cards*, with Gracie asleep next to me on the sofa, which I find calming. More often she chooses the chair next to Mark, and lies on her back with her black head hanging off the edge. I'm so glad we have her.

Wednesday 30 September

Good news, I think: one drain is down to 1 ml, so I ring Outra and she says come over to the hospital at lunchtime and she'll remove it. Before that, Mark and I take Gracie for a walk in the sunshine.

At the hospital, I lie on the bed as Outra and Mr Kothari chat away. As Outra removes the dressings, Mr Kothari examines me and acknowledges that the implant is standing 'proud' at the moment – which in normal circumstances might be an agreeable position for a breast, but when the other one doesn't match, it's not exactly model Eva Herzigová in her iconic 'Hello Boys' Wonderbra ad.

Up until this moment I haven't been able to see it because it's been covered with bandages, so I look down and see my own skin, breast-shaped, but higher up than the left side. I honestly don't mind the disparity at all, but Mr Kothari says we can't really judge for six months or so until it's settled.

Almost imperceptibly, Outra removes one of the drains by gently pulling it out of my skin and I barely feel a thing. She then asks how I'm getting on with the exercises.

'The exercises? What exercises?'

Somehow, of the dozens of booklets and literature I've been given to help prepare for the op, I've missed the one about what exercises to do immediately after a mastectomy to get yourself moving again. I'm cross at myself because I want to do everything I can to get back to normal as quickly as I can, when in fact I've missed a whole week in which I could have been improving my mobility.

Mr Kothari asks why I'm holding my arm at 90 degrees, and pulled in towards my stomach. I tell him it feels most comfortable like this. He challenges me to see if I can put my right arm through the sleeve of my shirt without help – and I can. How embarrassing. Maybe it's just my head that's been stopping me using it. As soon as I get home, I wash my hair, holding the shower head with my right hand. A small triumph.

Friday 2 October

Today I'm forty-seven years of age, and bloody hell, it feels good to be alive. Oliver, Joe and Mark bring presents and cards and tea into the bedroom and we all sit on the bed together as I unwrap my gifts. I am so grateful to be here, with my family, on my birthday, with the most significant part of my cancer treatment behind me. They've bought me a beautiful navy and white kimono dressing gown (I love anything Japanese), and a silver necklace with all their names engraved on it, including Gracie's. So beautiful, so thoughtful. I cry as I read some of the words Mark has written in his card to me. Ollie is filming me on my phone and stops as I begin getting upset. He'd never make a cameraman, I think, but I love him for his sensitivity.

At night Alex, Alexis and their girls, Paul, Cathy and their boys, John, Juliet and their son as well as Louisa come over and we chat, laugh, drink, eat and sing along to our favourite music. I appreciate these amazing people so much. All of them have helped our family in some way in the last couple of months – in practical terms by making food or ferrying the boys around, and emotionally, with kind texts or phone calls.

Louisa explains that some people ask her, 'How's Victoria?' and then follow it up with, 'And how are *you*?' She says it's like she has 'cancer by proxy'. Mark chips in with, 'Well, if Louisa's got cancer by proxy, then what must I have? Never mind you, Victoria, what about *us*? Maybe me and Louisa should record a video diary too.' It really makes us laugh.

And then there's the 'cancer card' Louisa has made me. Sometimes when I've asked for something recently (any-thing – could I have more time with this interviewee; are you getting the coffees in?), Louisa will say teasingly, 'Oh I get it, playing the cancer card, are we?' So she's taken an actual play-ing card from a deck, glued a picture of me on one side and written in black felt tip on the other: CANCER CARD. I put it in my back pocket and practise flourishing it, to the delight of everyone.

Alex brings a birthday cake she's made (her partner Alexis, meanwhile, brings more bags of home-made Bolognese sauce for me to put in the freezer), and when I blow out the candles, I make a wish. It's 'please don't let this cancer come back'. We raise our glasses, and as I look round at each of them – adults and kids – I say, 'Thank you to every single person in this room; each and every one of you stepped up. Thank you.' I mean every word.

Monday 5 October

I go to work today, not to return yet to presenting our pro-gramme, but to pre-record an interview with a member of Team GB, a race walker called Tom Bosworth. He's gay, and wants to come out on our programme. It's the only time he has free in his pre-Olympic training schedule, and I feel completely well (just a little self-conscious about the drains I'm carrying), so why not? It feels great to dress in smart work clothes and get back to doing what I love for a living: talking and listening to people.

Tom is absolutely lovely. We sit sideways on a sofa so I can hide the drains between me and the back of the couch where the camera won't be able to pick them up. He is friendly and articulate. We'll play the exclusive interview later in the week.

I pop in to see my boss, Keith, who's been a tower of strength, and I thank him for all the support and kindness he's shown me. We gossip about Robert Peston leaving the Beeb.

In the evening, Shelagh Fogarty, Elaine from work and Louisa come round and we have a laugh, a drink and a chat. They are brilliant company, which is why, I think, Joe joins us too until he goes to bed.

Wednesday 7 October

Mark and I go to see Mr Kothari to get all the facts about my tumour, and to find out if I'll need chemotherapy and radiotherapy. Mark's boss at Radio 2, Bob Shennan (he was also my old boss from 5 Live), has been incredibly supportive to us both, and work have been very flexible in allowing him the time to look after me and to be alongside me at these appointments. Outra's in the room, too, and Mark is poised with pen and notebook.

Mr Kothari begins, as he always does, by asking how I'm feeling. I reply, as I always do, with, 'Yep, I'm great, thank you, how are you?'

He then tells us about the tumour that he extracted just under two weeks ago.

'Firstly, the cancer has gone.'

It's incredible to hear those words.

'The tumour has been completely excised, and the area behind your nipple, which we preserved, is also free of cancer.'

I'm concentrating on his every word as Mark notes it all down.

'The size of the tumour was sixty-six millimetres.'

At which point I exclaim, 'Oh my God, that's double what we were initially told – bloody hell, how could I not have even spotted that?' I have hot tears in my eyes, and feel angry with myself. 'It's outrageous I didn't notice that.'

He talks about it being difficult to 'notice' because it wasn't a lump; it was diffused through the ducts of the breast. And he adds, 'Don't be harsh on yourself.'

He says it was a Grade 2 tumour (medium-growing), and had reached Stage 2B, which means it was over five centimetres and with a couple of lymph nodes 'touched'. There are four cancer stages: Stage 1 is the 'best', obviously, because it's likely to mean the cancer is small and hasn't moved anywhere else, and Stage 4 means it's spread.

As the tumour is 66 mm, it's 'just beyond the threshold for radiotherapy, which is five centimetres'. I don't understand why we're using millimetres and centimetres, but that's the least of my worries. What I'm focusing on is the knowledge that I *will* be having radiotherapy and that I'm not entirely sure what it is, but before I can ask, Mr Kothari continues:

'And it's likely you'll be having chemotherapy, but that's down to the oncologist, who you will see in a couple of weeks.'

OK, so I'm having chemo too.

As I take all this in he catches the expression of realisation on my face and says, in a matter-of-fact way, 'But you're not afraid of anything.'

I'm not, he's right; but it's a lot of information to absorb and it's going to take time to process it. We thank him and Outra again and then end up having a jovial chat about the respective leadership skills of managers in the NHS and the BBC.

On the drive home, we discuss what we now know about the cancer. I'm suspicious about the Stage 2B bit – surely there's a Stage 2 and a Stage 3, and if I'm not Stage 2, I must be a Stage 3. But it's gone, and that's the most important thing, Mark reminds me. As for chemotherapy and radiotherapy, I feel flat about those. I need to work it through in my head and rationalise it, and can't at the moment.

I email Keith at work to update him about the prospect of further treatment and he replies quite reasonably, 'And this is what you were expecting, so it's all good?' He's right, of course, but I haven't yet been able to come to the same conclusion.

Thursday 8 October

I catch the train to Waterloo to meet my mum, who's coming down from Bolton to stay. On the concourse I call Alex and end up weeping down the phone to her, desperate and indignant. I feel sorry for the bloke sitting next to me, who can hear me telling my sister I'm angry about having to have chemotherapy and that I don't want it to be depressing and miserable. She listens, is sympathetic but in the end she says, 'But it is the right thing.'

So far, remarkably, this experience has been much more positive than I ever in a million years could have hoped for, but the stories you hear about the effects of chemo – losing your hair, chronic fatigue, loss of motivation – it's just not me, and I don't want to feel like that. Plus I also don't understand why, when I expected I would be needing chemo, and in fact wanted it, because it reduces the chances of the cancer recurring, I'm not embracing it – or at least confronting it, as I have done so far with everything I've faced in this process. I feel guilty too; I should be grateful to be having chemo – it's an option not offered to some cancer patients because their illness has progressed too far.

I don't tell my mum about my worries, although I suspect she can tell I've been crying. Meanwhile I think Mark's running on empty.

Friday 9 October

My mum does loads of jobs around the house: ironing, cleaning, the lot. We talk about how I'm feeling about chemo. I know I want to work as much as I can through it, but what I definitely don't want is people turning on the TV to watch our programme and being distracted from the story we're covering by my loss of hair or me wearing a scarf round my head. And the only way round that is to get a wig. There's no other solution, as far as I can see, so I have to accept it.

My mum asks how we think the boys are doing. Pretty robust, pragmatic and normal, we reply, but we can't know for certain. When we ask them how they are, they always say they're OK and glad the operation is in the past. But who knows, long term? Their day-to-day behaviour is, broadly speaking, good, and they seem as sociable and outgoing as they have always been.

When Joe gets home I check if he *is* OK and ask if anyone's said anything to him at school. He reports that a girl in his class asked him if his mum had cancer, to which he apparently replied, 'Yes, but it's not real cancer, because she's not going to die.' I smile and explain to him that it is real cancer, but having cancer doesn't necessarily mean you're going to die, particularly as the doctors and nurses are so brilliant these days at treating it. He accepts that, nods and carries on making a snack.

Monday 12 October

A clip from my first video diary went online last night as a trail ahead of the full film being shown on BBC 2 this morning, and when I look at Facebook and Twitter, I can see hundreds and hundreds of tremendous messages from followers, viewers, Radio 5 Live listeners, cancer patients, breast cancer survivors, NHS staff and others. I cannot believe the reaction – I was not expecting this at all. People are telling me it's touched them, moved them – they describe it as 'honest', 'inspiring', 'remarkable' and say it will help women facing the same challenge.

At 9.15 a.m. my mum and I sit down and watch my film about having a mastectomy go out on our TV programme. It's surreal. She has tears in her eyes, and my brother Nick emails to say it made him cry. I'm overwhelmed by the reaction from everyone, and it has the immediate effect of making me feel subdued, I think because I hadn't prepared for this kind of feedback. And there's also a small part of my brain that still won't accept this is happening to me.

In the afternoon I travel into London to meet Louisa at Westminster. On the train a middle-aged man is reading a copy of the *Telegraph* with a large photo of me on the front above quotes from my video diary. I slink away from him because I feel embarrassed. Louisa tells me the quantity and quality of the comments from viewers in response to the diary is astonishing, and that it has featured in every national newspaper, making the front of the *Telegraph*, *Daily Mail* and *Mirror*.

We attend a portrait exhibition at the House of Commons I've been invited to, featuring tasteful and bold photographs of women who've had mastectomies. As we queue to go through security, the guard asks me to place the small handbag that's slung across me diagonally onto the conveyor belt so it can be checked. I pause and worry and say rather pathetically, 'I need this bag for medical reasons' (my drains are hidden inside).

'I'm sorry, madam, I need you to place it on here so we can scan it.'

'I understand,' I say, embarrassed, and from nowhere my eyes start to fill with tears. I don't want to have to remove the drains and the plastic pouch filled with blood in front of everyone, which is completely illogical because I've filmed them and put the footage online and broadcast it on national television. Louisa overhears and briefly explains and the security guard immediately gets it; I show him discreetly what's in the bag and he waves me on.

A Conservative MP called Chloe Smith gives a short speech and says how pleased she is that such an important record of breast cancer surgery is being featured in the heart of Westminster. I'm only there because I too share something in common with these women featured in the exhibition. Afterwards, Louisa and I decide to explore Parliament and end up trying to get into the terrace bar – it's empty, though, so we leave, and then head up to the public gallery to watch politicians in action in the Commons chamber. We arrive at a particularly dramatic time: Labour's Deputy Leader, Tom Watson, is in full flow, explaining why he won't be apologising for demanding the police investigate sexual abuse claims against the late Lord Brittan. It's the first time I've ever been here, and looking down, it feels like I'm observing actors in a play that's reached a particularly tense, electric moment.

A short piece about my diary appears on the BBC's six o'clock news. I can't believe it's getting so much coverage.

Tuesday 13 October

The *Daily Mail* and the *Sun* transcribe some of my video footage and feature it in their editions today. James Harding texts to tell me he thought it was 'amazing'. *Guardian* columnist Deborah Orr writes a comment piece suggesting I've 'oversimplified' breast cancer. Her criticism stings because she might be spot on – I have no idea. It's simply how I approached the illness.

I make an appointment at the wig shop for tomorrow, and because of a suggestion from Keith, I call his former colleague from *The Times*, Anne Spackman, who's recently had cancer, to talk about hair loss. It's empowering talking to others who've had this disease because it encourages you to think, if they did it, I can do it. She tells me that a combination of the chemo drug she was on for her type of breast cancer (Taxol), plus wearing a cold cap helped preserve most of her hair. The cap works by narrowing the blood vessels just beneath the skin of the scalp, reducing the amount of chemo that reaches the hair follicles – hence more chance of keeping your hair. She recommends some expensive shampoo (Pureology), and generally gives me encouragement and strength for the next part of the treatment. I am so grateful to her.

Wednesday 14 October

It's utterly surreal to come downstairs with the boys to see *Good Morning Britain* hosts Kate Garraway and Susanna Reid asking their guest Gloria Hunniford about my video diary, and whether being public about a cancer diagnosis helps others. Gloria's daughter, Caron Keating, died aged forty-one after being diagnosed with breast cancer. I feel apprehensive about how she's going to answer the question. My film is so personal and yet so out there, exactly as I wanted it to be, but I wasn't prepared for my approach to the illness to be debated in this way. Ms Hunniford says some very kind things about how I'm dealing with it, adding that she believes it really does help when people are open because it encourages others to check their breasts, or seek treatment, and it breaks down the taboo of talking about cancer.

The final drain is being removed today. Hurray! It's another step forward in the process, and means I can go back to presenting the programme again soon, full-time. Mr Kothari and Outra chat to me about my video diary, and both express the view that it will definitely help others who are going through breast cancer. It's gratifying to have the support of medical professionals.

Outra extracts the second drain, and then it dawns on me that this bit of being looked after by Mr Kothari and Outra is over: it's goodbye, because now I'll be handed into the care of an oncologist. I shake Mr Kothari's hand and tell him I can never, ever, ever thank him enough. He smiles and leaves the room, and I start crying in front of Outra and tell her I don't want to not see them again. She hugs me and tells me I can come and visit them any time.

Then she looks at me with tears in her eyes and says, 'You know, you have been a star patient. Some people when they're told they have cancer shut down, whereas you have concentrated on living, rather than on the cancer. You should be very proud of yourself.' I cry even more. I love this woman.

In the afternoon I spend an hour and a half in the company of Amy Holt, the lady who makes wigs. She is young (thirty-ish, I'd say), petite, well spoken and with an extremely kind, gentle nature. I cannot believe how many considerate people I've met in the last couple of months. We sit in a cosy top-floor boutique-type room, her salon, above an estate agents' in Richmond. On the back wall are mannequin heads made of white polystyrene, and resting on top of each one is a wig in a variety of hair colours. I sit at her glass table with a large mirror in front of me and we talk about her work – she makes wigs for women who lose their hair through chemo and through alopecia and for women who just prefer to wear wigs. I confess that the idea of me wearing a wig is pretty horrific because I associate them with elderly ladies, and I also think everyone can tell when someone's wearing a wig, but that in order to continue presenting my programme, I need one so it won't detract from the content. Amy explains that her wigs are made of human hair so they move naturally, and with a proper fitting and choosing the right colours, no one will know. I worry about how long it will take to fix it on each morning in the early hours before going to work, how I'll wash it, dry it and style it, and how I'll stop it flying off. She smiles, and says she knows I won't believe her right now, but I will be able to put it on securely in just a few minutes once I get into the habit, and it won't, repeat won't, ever come off. She's right, I don't believe her, but she says it so confidently, I am willing to try.

She begins to measure my head so she can make a wig that fits. This involves tying my shoulder-length hair back into a low, tight ponytail before covering my head in cling film, which she Sellotapes down. This takes about fifteen minutes. As she removes it, I can see it's going to be the mould for the lace cap to which human hair will be attached. She places the cling film cap on a mannequin head.

Then she brings to the table about twenty bunches of shiny, soft, real hair, each about a foot long, that are similar to the colour of my own hair – light brown, with blonder bits in it (that's twenty years of highlights).

'Whose hair *is* this? It's beautiful,' I ask suspiciously.

Amy explains that she sources it from a number of suppliers across Europe, and that women donate or sell it.

I rather enjoy choosing the bunches of hair that will be sewn to the lace cap that will make my wig: it's a challenge to find a combination that will look like the colour of my natural hair. I wasn't expecting there'd be so much choice.

It will take Amy around six weeks to make the wig. I don't know if I'll need it by then, but it's good to be prepared.

Thursday 15 October

We've known for some time that Mark's facing redundancy. Because of the cancer, we haven't worried about it for ages. Perspective is all. Today he's meeting Mark Goodier, the boss of an independent production company called Wise Buddah, to talk about doing some work for him, hopefully, in the future. It's not a formal interview, just a chat. I really hope he gets some good news, because he deserves it.

I log into my BBC email from home, and there are more wonderful messages to reply to from people who used to listen to me on Radio 5 Live and from people who watch our programme. Many say they too are about to have a mastectomy, and that watching my video diary has not only inspired them, but it's 'taken away their fear'. Taken away their fear? I am utterly astounded. I never expected, ever, that one of the effects of talking about cancer and explaining what a mastectomy can involve would be to reduce the debilitating anxiety others were facing. I simply thought that showing the practical aspects of what the surgery involved might be useful information to put into the public domain. If that's the result, then it's been worth it.

Via direct messages on Twitter, I've been talking to Jacquie Beltrao, who presents the sport on Sky News each morning. She contacted me immediately after I posted that I had breast cancer to say that she'd listened to me for years on the radio on her journey home from work each morning, and felt like she knew me. She had breast cancer a couple of years ago, and urges me to call her if I ever need any help. Today I speak to her and she is lovely. We talk about how we both are, and she tells me she took six months off work for her chemotherapy, and what her diet now consists of: she's given up all dairy and red meat because it makes her feel better, but she still drinks wine. Hurray! Talking to people who've had breast cancer and are through the other side is very, very comforting.

When I collect Mark from the station, he is buoyant. The meeting, he says, has been very encouraging, but then, as we both acknowledge, he's had encouraging meetings before and it hasn't led to getting work. But it definitely lifts us, and then when Ollie gets home and announces he has no homework tonight, well, it seems like we should celebrate. Post-surgery, I feel like celebrating everything, because life actually *is* too short, so why not? We go out for tea to the local pub.

Louisa forwards me various requests for interviews from newspapers, magazines and ITV shows like *Good Morning Britain* and *Lorraine*, which I decline. It feels as though I've said everything in the video diary.

Friday 16 October

Mark Goodier asks Mark to work on an interview series that Wise Buddah will make for Radio 2!! It's brilliant news, and suddenly feels like one less thing to worry about.

I write to Gloria Hunniford, via her agent, to thank her for her compassionate comments on TV the other day.

Saturday 17 October

On BBC1 on a Saturday morning at about a quarter to eight there's a programme called *Newswatch*. It's like *Points of View*, but solely about news programmes. As I'm making the boys' porridge, I hear the presenter referring to the viewer who's written in to complain that there should have been a warning before an excerpt of my video diary showing the after-effects of my surgery was broadcast on the BBC's 6 p.m. news bulletin last Monday. I'm mildly flabbergasted. A warning about what? Skin being exposed? The sight of bandages? The very fact of talking about a mastectomy? The viewer didn't elaborate. As my grandma used to say, there's nowt so strange as folk.

Sunday 18 October

I'm finding it hard to relax. Tomorrow we meet the oncologist to talk about the next stage of treatment – chemotherapy. I don't have enough facts yet about why I need it, what the odds are of the cancer returning with and without it and what the side effects are. I delve into the Sunday papers to try to distract my mind.

Monday 19 October

Mark and I meet Dr Teoh, the oncologist, for the first time. Yet again another clever, efficient, compassionate health profession-al. With her is Regina, a breast cancer nurse, who I later ascertain is from the Philippines. Dr Teoh quietly talks us through what she has learned about my cancer and how treatment should proceed from here. Mark is ready with his notebook.

She explains that what was not in my favour was the size of the tumour; what was in my favour was the fact that the can-cer was ER-positive – oestrogen-positive, which means it can respond well to hormonal therapies. 'ER' is used because the American spelling of oestrogen is estrogen. My cancer is also HER2-negative, she tells us (it stands for human epidermal growth factor receptor 2, and as it's negative, it's not relevant to my illness). HER2 is a gene that, if it's not working correctly, can play a role in breast cancer. She adds that HER2-positive breast cancers tend to be more aggressive.

She continues: even though two of the lymph nodes were touched by microscopic bits of cancer (officially called micro-metastases), she is approaching my cancer as 'node-negative' because the cancer cells were so minute, and therefore she rec-ommends six sessions of chemotherapy to eliminate any cancer cells that may or may not be elsewhere in my body.

Dr Teoh speaks clearly and logically and I understand everything.

I think out loud.

'What if we approach the cancer as node-positive, what differ-ence would it make?'

She says it would involve more aggressive drugs, and would bring down, by another 3 to 4 per cent, the chances of it recurring within ten years.

She goes on, 'Without any further treatment, the chances of the cancer coming back are twenty to thirty per cent. Chemotherapy reduces it by another third. Radiotherapy by another five per cent, and the more ferocious chemo regime by another three to four per cent.'

Swiftly, both Mark and I do the maths.

'OK, for the sake of it, let's take the worst-case scenario,' I (predictably) say. 'Thirty per cent chance of it coming back with no further treatment. A third off for chemo – that's down to twenty per cent.'

Mark: 'Then radiotherapy takes off five per cent, so we're now at fifteen per cent, and with the more aggressive regime taking off another three or four per cent, we're down to eleven to twelve per cent. So there's around a one in ten chance of it coming back in the next decade.'

'It's gonna be me, isn't it?' I suggest drily.

Mark, exasperated and yet still kind: 'Or you're going to be in the ninety per cent who don't get it again!'

We talk briefly about the pros and cons of going for the node-negative or node-positive approach, and although it's not said explicitly, it's clear that it's my choice, which again surprises and delights me because it helps me feel empowered.

It seems like a no-brainer to me to go for node-positive, because the potential side effects will be pretty similar. Dr Teoh says that's absolutely fine, no problem, then talks us through the drugs I'll be given – FEC-T, pronounced 'fec-tee'. The first three sessions feature fluorouracil, epirubicin and cyclophosphamide, and for the final three sessions I'll be given docetaxel, also known by its registered name as Taxotere, hence the 'T'. The combination of these drugs should kill any stray cancer cells left in my body. There are three weeks between each cycle (in my head I calculate that it's eighteen weeks in total – four and a bit months, so I'll be done by February 2016).

She addresses the main side effects of chemo – sickness, aches and pains and possible hair loss – in a matter-of-fact way, and says she'll give me drugs to try to alleviate all of those. She makes it really clear that she and the staff will do all they can to make it as pain-free as possible. I tell her I want to work through chemo, and she says I must do whatever I want to do that helps me feel better. Dr Teoh hands me a printed sheet from Macmillan Cancer Support on the effects of the FEC-T regime. I scan the list: woah, there are twenty-seven possible side effects, ranging from the common – hair loss, feeling sick, bruising and bleeding, diarrhoea, to the less common – blood clot risk, changes in the way the heart works, fertility issues.

We talk about when I should start, and I get out my work diary. It could be 28 October, but looking ahead I realise that would mean the second session would be three days before Paul's fortieth, and I'm not missing that. So if we push it back a week, to 2 November, I will have got over the first session, be able to go to the party and have the second lots of drugs the Wednesday after the do. Result. Dr Teoh is happy with that. Before we leave, I ask where she was born; Malaysia, she tells us, and has been in the UK for twenty-one years.

When I text Natalie to let her know which drugs I'm going to be having, she says she had exactly the same, and she managed to get through OK. Plus, she said, you don't get anywhere near even half the side effects printed on the list.

Just over three weeks ago I was getting my clothes ready for going into hospital. Now I'm ironing clothes to wear on my programme tomorrow. I can't wait to go back to work.

Tuesday 20 October

It's 1.30 a.m. and I'm awake, thinking about chemotherapy. I can't really imagine what it'll be like or how it's going to affect me. I'm considering wearing the cold cap – the thing that looks like a jockey's hat that freezes your head while you're having chemo in order to help preserve your hair. I've heard awful stories about it, but if it means keeping your hair, or some of it, I'm definitely going to try it. And if I'm one of the ones for whom the cold cap works, I won't really need the wig after all.

The routine of going into work feels reassuringly normal – getting up early, letting Gracie out for a wee, reading the papers on the way in, saying hi to the security guards in BBC reception. And, pleasingly, everyone is the same; there are the same laughs, the same irritations, and when the programme begins I feel confident and ready to go, particularly as I have no pain at all from surgery last month.

There are many 'welcome back' messages on Twitter, and I receive a lovely one from Sarah Montague, a BBC colleague from Radio 4, who says she is pleased to see me at work again, and that 'your reporting on yourself was absolutely gripping, couldn't turn away. And also reassuring xx'.

In the office are dozens of cards from well-wishers who watch our programme and saw the video diary. There's only one that talks about someone they know dying from breast cancer.

Wednesday 21 October

It's the *PinkNews* Awards tonight, being held at the Foreign and Commonwealth Office, and it's my first night out since having surgery. I'm very happy and up for some fun. We're nominated in the Broadcaster of the Year category, alongside various other network radio and TV journalists and shows. *PinkNews* is, according to their Twitter handle, 'the world's most read LGBT+ digital media publisher'. Our coverage of stories since we launched in April includes an exclusive story featuring two of the youngest transgender children in Britain, aged six and eight, in which we revealed figures of how many under-tens were being treated by the NHS's only clinic dedicated to identity issues (picked up by all the national press), and Tom Bosworth coming out a few weeks ago. We're in fantastic moods, enhanced by a glass of pink champagne being handed to us as we arrive in the stunningly beautiful Victorian atrium of the Foreign Office, decorated with dramatic and elegant gilt coving and murals on its vast ceiling. And then we win it! We are so delighted, and I make a short speech thanking the readers of *PinkNews* who voted for us and say I hope we've created a trusted environment on our programme where people feel they can talk about really important stuff.

Various MPs chat to us, a number saying they thought my video diary was 'amazing', which is very kind. I spot an actress I recognise from the brilliant *Boy Meets Girl* on BBC2, so introduce myself – she's Rebecca Root, one of Britain's very few transgender actresses. Then Alex Salmond stops me to congratulate me on my first day back at work after surgery (he read it in the papers this morning), and I thank him and ask him if he knows Rhona Cameron (who is the awards' host) and would he be so kind as to introduce all of us to her, please? He happily obliges, and Rebecca, Rhona, Louisa and I start chatting away as Mr Salmond tries to get a word in.

Thursday 22 October

I receive a brief email from Mr Kothari in the evening:

> Watched your programmes last 2 days, very good – proud of you.
> BW
> Manish Kothari

I'm genuinely pleased he's taken the time to check on me via the medium of TV!

Friday 23 October

I can't get out of my head that the cancer in me is going to come back. That it just will. I don't want to be miserable or pessimistic or depressing; I just fear that it will.

An email from a friend lifts me, entitled 'Thought you'd like to hear this'.

Hi,

This morning I went to have a mammogram at the Lady McAdden Centre in Southend http://www.ladymcaddenbreastunit.co.uk/

It's a charity and I've been going there since Mum was diagnosed with breast cancer. Although I'm now 50 (!) and qualify for the NHS screening programme it might not kick in for another three years and the good thing about the unit is you book yourself in and you don't have to wait long for an appointment. The other really good thing is they ask for a donation but if you have no money that's fine, you still get screened.

Anyway, I'm chatting away – to avoid the obvious (there I am with no top on!) – and the nurse says they've been extra busy – because of you, Victoria. The last time they saw a spike like this was when Kylie Minogue was diagnosed. So then I said I knew you and she said how the whole unit had watched your film and how they thought about asking you to be a patron but figured you'd be inundated with requests. She also said that your young

age has prompted many younger women to be in contact. I said
I was sure you'd be really pleased to hear that – you are, aren't
you? Didn't want to put words in your mouth!

Anyway have a restful weekend after your busy week. Zoe was
16 last Monday and we're off to Chiquito's!!

Love Nicky xx

I am absolutely stunned, I really am. And humbled. And so delighted. Wow. Plus it's the first time I've ever been mentioned in
the same breath as Kylie (and the last, no doubt). If women are
going to get themselves checked, that is brilliant.

We go round to friends that night, Vicky and Steve, who we
met through Oliver's old football team. There are eight of us
and we have such a laugh. One of the dads, Phil, is there with
his new (ish) partner, Debbie, who is good fun. Phil's wife died
of breast cancer three years ago. Mark, the boys and I attended
her funeral. After everyone asks me how I'm doing, we crack on
with the evening.

Cathy and Paul come back to ours after for a late drink, and
I get upset talking to Cathy about my fears that the cancer will
return. She envelops me with hugs and tries to encourage me
to stop thinking like that. Then she urges me to go and get my
diary, so she can work out when the chemo cycles are and book
lovely things for us to do in between – like tickets to see Hozier,
who I love.

Saturday 24 October

I talk to Mark about the imaginary scene that's in my head: Mark is on a night out with Cathy, Paul, Phil, Debbie, Vicky and Steve – everyone who was there last night. Mark is with someone, anyone – but not me, though, because I'm dead. And around him people are saying, 'Oh, Mark, you look so happy,' just like we were saying to Phil last night. I cry about this as I tell him and bury my head in his chest. He wraps me in a hug and tries to comfort me by saying, first, I am not going to die; and secondly, the idea that that would happen when I have been such a huge part of his life, when his life has been defined by me, is absurd. I cry like a child does when they start to lose their breath, and simply can't stop sobbing.

Allowing my mind to think like this is destructive, I know. It's a totally unproductive worry. I need to work this image through in my head and get rid of it. I try to convince myself of this: if I think the cancer might return (and, obviously, I don't know that it's going to), then I have to think, equally, that it might not return (because I don't know that it's going to). I remind myself of the percentage chance of it recurring – it's about 11 to 12 per cent. That's OK. It could be so much worse. I am one of the lucky ones.

Mark and the boys go off to see West Ham, so it's Gracie and me hanging out together for the day. It's peaceful and perfect. On a dog walk I bump into a neighbour and we stop and chat. He tells me about his friend who's mid-fifties who recently discovered a tumour in his stomach, 'and he went to get it checked out and three months later he was dead'.

I'm stunned into silence for a heartbeat as I absorb what he's telling me. Then wonder why he's saying this out loud.

'Oh my goodness, I am so sorry to hear that; what a shock it must have been. I'm so, so sorry,' I say, before swiftly getting away to continue my walk.

West Ham beat Chelsea, therefore Oliver, Joe and Mark are in great moods when they arrive home, and their presence helps me forget the conversation with the neighbour.

Louisa sends me a photo of Amanda Platell's column in the *Daily Mail* today where she writes:

> Returning to work less than a month after having a mastectomy, Victoria Derbyshire is an inspiration, not just to those with breast cancer but to anyone with a serious illness. Hope is the greatest companion during such times, and her courage – filming her treatment to be shown on TV – was awesome to behold.
>
> Yet I think we should also spare a thought for others with cancer who may not be as strong as Victoria, nor as supported by family and friends. Not everyone will be back to normal life in a short time and no one should feel that if they can't make a speedy recovery, somehow they've failed.
>
> As Victoria said, everyone's experience is different – and hers was honestly and bravely told. But I hope she knows also that no one will think less of her, if, in a few weeks' time, the lure of her family and her home proves greater than the studio for a while.

She's right – each of us as cancer patients has to find our own way. That might be sharing our experiences, or not; it might be taking time off work, or not; it might be trying to be positive when you feel you can and accepting it when you can't. There's no right or wrong way to deal with cancer; it's whatever works for you.

Sunday 25 October

I wake up feeling much more constructive and ready to get on with the chemo. If it wasn't for the hair loss, chemotherapy really would be OK, I reckon. But what do I know, never having experienced it?

We visit Ben and Natalie at their new house in Kent. I ask Natalie about the recovery times during each three-week cycle, and the cold cap. She tells me that on the Sunday after her very first session – so five days after FEC-T was pumped into her system – she was out having lunch and drinking wine with her mum. I'm impressed. It gives me enormous encouragement, but she adds that with each cycle you do become more tired. She advises that I plan nothing for the first seven days after chemo except sleeping, then if I want to, I could go back to work until the next session. She wanted to work through her treatment, but her former employer took the decision to sign her off sick, which she found totally disempowering. I was shocked a boss could do that, but they told her she was a 'risk to them'. Who did she work for? A charity.

She reveals that the hardest thing for her was losing her hair. She tried the cold cap for a couple of sessions, but some of her hair fell out anyway so she gave up on it. Eventually she asked her hairdresser to shave it all off.

'How cold is the cold cap?' I enquire.

'Freezing, absolutely freezing, and it gives you a headache and can make you feel sick, but you do get used to it after a while.'

She tells me about avoiding picking up infections. Chemo causes your infection-fighting white blood cells to decrease, which means you're vulnerable to getting coughs, colds, the lot, from anyone. It can lead to you being admitted to hospital with a high temperature and possible sepsis, which can be fatal. It all sounds overly dramatic to me, but who am I to argue? She recalls how Ben had a bad cold during her chemo, and she was effectively quarantined in their bedroom. He would bring her a meal on a tray, leave it outside the door and she would only emerge to take the tray when he was back downstairs.

'But,' she says, 'it's all doable.'

Even armed with all this factual information, I'm incredibly apprehensive. It's fear of the unknown. I want to get the first one under my belt, then I'll know what I'm dealing with. It reminds me of how I felt at school waiting to take an A-level exam – a heavy brick of dread in the pit of my stomach.

Natalie asks in a charmingly roundabout way if I'll consider being an ambassador for the new charity she works for – YouCan (Youth Cancer), for ten- to twenty-nine-year-olds whose lives have been affected by cancer. It's so roundabout, I actually have to check if that is what she *is* asking me! I feel honoured, and my first question is, 'What does an ambassador do?'

Monday 26 October

Actress Rebecca Root is on the programme today to respond to Germaine Greer's view that transgender women 'aren't women'. Ms Root is eloquent, understated yet passionate. Ms Greer declined to give us an interview, but in a statement to us says this: 'Just because you lop off your penis and then wear a dress doesn't make you a f****** woman,' adding, 'I've asked my doctor to give me long ears and liver spots and I'm going to wear a brown coat, but that won't turn me into a f****** cocker spaniel.' Rebecca's shocked laughter when I read her this statement says it all: Germaine Greer's view is offensive to trans women, and the way she's expressed her view in this statement is outrageous.

The government's cuts to tax credits is the main story today, though, a huge issue for our audience.

I receive an email asking me to open a new research centre at UCL that is trying to find a cure for breast cancer.

Tuesday 27 October

The boys, Mark and I go to meet Emma, a nurse in the 'Infusion Suite' at Ashford Hospital. The word 'infusion' has gentle, relaxing, positive connotations for me, so I look up the medical definition on my phone and it says, 'the slow therapeutic introduction of fluid other than blood into the vein'.

This is my pre-chemotherapy assessment, and I'm keen the boys meet the staff and see the place where I'll be coming to spend one morning every three weeks until February. It means, I hope, that by seeing the reality, their imaginations won't allow them to conjure up some dark, frightening place. They've heard the word 'chemotherapy' a lot in recent weeks, and probably have little idea of what it means. I want them to hear some facts.

Emma is warm and smiling and welcomes us into the Infusion Suite which is bright, light and airy. We like her immediately. She's young (thirty-ish), down to earth, confident and she's got cheeky eyes – I bet she's a laugh on a night out. She directs me to sit in one of the large blue comfy armchairs that remind me of the kind my grandparents used to have in their front room, the ones where the bottom part swings upward to support your legs. Mark and the boys pull up a couple of seats too, and Emma talks us through what will happen next Wednesday, my first session. Effectively I will sit there for a couple of hours while drugs are injected into a cannula that will be attached to the top of my left hand (avoiding the right side, because I use that the most). She runs through the side effects in a factual way and says that they will give me a steroid a day in the three days running up to the morning itself, and some painkillers to take after, which, even if I'm feeling OK, I must take. The steroids should stop the drugs from making me vomit. She talks about the risks of picking up an infection and that we must all make sure we wash our hands regularly, or even better, keep plenty of small bottles of hand sanitiser around the house. Plus I need to buy a thermometer in case my temperature does rise. If it goes over 37.5 degrees, then I need to get myself swiftly to A&E. She gives me a debit-card-sized leaflet with the following words printed on the front: INFORMATION FOR ACCIDENT & EMERGENCY STAFF: the patient is receiving chemotherapy and has a high risk of developing neutropenic sepsis, which is a MEDICAL EMERGENCY.

If I ever need to go to A&E with a temperature, it's what I hand straight over to the staff there. It all sounds a bit apocalyptic.

'And of course, boys, while your mum's having chemo, it means you'll have to do all the jobs around the house, and' (she looks at me and her eyes twinkle) 'it means your dad can't drink any alcohol at all!' The two of them think this is hilarious, and with that one line, Emma cleverly makes us all feel relaxed.

I ask her, if she was about to embark on chemo, would she wear a cold cap?

She's emphatic.

'No. I've seen too many women disappointed because it hasn't worked.'

I'm glad she's honest, but I feel crushed. I tell her I'm not really expecting it to work, I just want to try it.

As we're leaving, we realise the Infusion Suite has Wi-Fi. They really have thought of everything.

Wednesday 28 October

It amazes me that I can joke about having a mastectomy, but I do. I suppose it's because the op went OK, the scar is healing well and I've got full mobility back in my right arm. Plus, black humour can be therapeutic at times. Louisa and I are in the studio preparing for the programme, with Dickie, one of our finest floor managers, who also happens to be good fun. He's asking me how I'm doing, and for some reason it occurs to me to ask him if he can tell which side I had the mastectomy on. He steps back a few paces, takes a brief look at my chest and says, 'I'm a gay man – of course I can tell, it's the right side.' We collapse in hysterics.

Sunday 1 November

I'm impatient. I want chemotherapy to begin. I really do need to crack on with this now, so I know what I'm dealing with. I ask Mark how he's feeling about it.

'It's a huge investment in the future of our family.' He's right. With chemotherapy, my chances of living a longer life are immeasurably boosted. My chances of seeing my boys grow into decent young men, watching them marry, have children of their own . . . it's that thought I need to hold on to.

Monica from work texts me to say her friend has had chemo, and she recommends wearing dark nail varnish throughout because it successfully preserved her nails. I love Monica for all sorts of reasons, but especially for passing this advice on and make a mental note to paint my nails black before Wednesday. It's worth a try.

Monday 2 November

I want the next two days to go quickly. At work I'm apprehensive and edgy, and I'm finding it hard to speak properly to anyone. I can't concentrate, and I just want to be with Mark and the boys. Once home, I take Gracie out for a long walk, which is a calming distraction. She's a magnificent addition to our family at a very challenging time.

Tuesday 3 November

It's one of those early mornings at work where we're on the back foot from the start. Fresh stories that have broken overnight need chasing, fixing, writing, and I need to read up on them too. We catch up, though, and the programme goes OK. As I dash home, Keith rings to give me courage for tomorrow. 'You have looked this thing in the eye, confronted it head-on, now keep going,' he tells me. My mum calls, as do Nick and Alex, and Anna. I collect together all the things I'm going to need over the hours the drugs are being injected into me: water, my diary, *Homes & Gardens* magazine, *House & Garden* magazine, *BBC Homes & Antiques* magazine, the GoPro camera, a fabric headband (like I used at ballet, aged five, but this one's black, not pale pink) to wear under the cold cap, where it will shield the edge of my face from the ice, a scarf and my mobile.

Alan, a super-talented hairdresser who's been cutting my hair for twenty years, comes over to ceremoniously take two and a half inches off the length of it, as recommended by nurse Emma. She says the longer and heavier the hair is, the more it might be likely to pull and fall out. He's brilliantly upbeat and encouraging, as always, and suggests I wear my favourite clothes tomorrow. I say I don't think a cold cap will go well with my red D&G dress, somehow, but the black nail varnish will look good, at least.

Wednesday 4 November

The day is finally here. I'm not afraid, but I am agitated, because I don't know what it involves, and I want it out of the way. Mark and I arrive at the Infusion Suite promptly at 9 a.m., and Emma asks where I'd like to sit. I choose a corner, the big armchair seat next to a bed with a window on each wall. Light and cosy; if a hospital ward that administers chemotherapy which kills all your cells can ever be cosy. Emma switches on the cumbersome cooling machine, the size of a small fridge, alongside me that is attached to the cold cap, which isn't yet cold, via a large plastic tube. It all seems terribly low-tech for the twenty-first century.

I have to put the cap on half an hour before the chemotherapy drugs are administered. The red and black head garment is heavier than you'd imagine, and ugly, and it feels as though it's made of the same rubbery fabric as a wetsuit. Immediately underneath the rubber cap are plastic tubes coiled in a circle, into which the cooling solution is pumped. It has to get down to −3 degrees before it goes on my head. Shit. Not even zero is enough; it has to be a minus number. As we wait, Emma in her rubber gloves puts conditioner all over my dry hair as further protection and to smooth it flat, and I then place the headband around the edge of my face and Emma tries to fit the cap on. It's awkward, and we have to pull it down roughly so it actually does touch the top of my head. A black strap under my chin keeps it in place. It's a shock because it's bloody cold, and I instinctively tremble and shake my head as though trying to unsettle the chill that's descending on me. It's like washing your hair in freezing cold water. Deeply unpleasant. Yet within a few minutes, I acclimatise, and it gradually begins to feel OK, which astonishes me.

Emma sits by me and fixes a cannula in the top of my left hand, a small plastic tube into which the syringe containing the drugs will fit, and I take an anti-sickness tablet (a steroid) in preparation. Mark is opposite me, checking I'm OK, asking if I want a newspaper or his iPad. Focusing to read when your head is frozen is hard, but I'm glad I do. The chief sports writer of the *Telegraph*, Paul Hayward, has very unusually written a piece about his own treatment for a type of head and neck cancer, and how having the goal of covering a home rugby World Cup gave him something to aim for as he was enduring some particularly ferocious treatment.

The piece is magnificent, thoughtful, but most of all optimistic. During his treatment he took joy from some wonderful athletes.

> Then came the sharpest ray of light. Barcelona v Bayern Munich at Camp Nou, in May. On the screen in a room short on cheer, Lionel Messi collected a pass on his left foot, turned inside then out in an impossibly narrow channel and sent Jérôme Boateng, the Bayern defender, falling sideways like a felled tree. Out came Manuel Neuer, the world's best goalkeeper, to quash the threat with a giant, raised arm. And Messi chipped him. Chipped one of the biggest and most intimidating men in football.

> As the ball bounced into the net Rafinha, another Bayern defender, went with it, his body a tangle of thwarted desperation. The camera panned round the crowd to capture the sense of wonder. A man in an Argentina shirt and Barcelona scarf was having a religious experience. On the commentary, Martin Tyler said: 'Only football can make you feel like this.' I felt myself rise from my chair, and illness fell away.

'Illness fell away.' I can't wait for that to happen to me. What an evocative, inspiring phrase. His column is stunning, and I message him on Twitter to tell him.

Soon thirty minutes is up, and I'm about to have chemotherapy drugs for the first time. Emma takes a large syringe and, through the cannula, begins to inject the first solution of colourless drugs into me. All I feel is a slight cooling sensation on the top of my hand, and that's it.

I don't think I'd realised until this moment that Emma would be sitting with me the whole time. I'd imagined the drugs would have been administered from a drip. Maybe I've just seen that on TV.

Emma gets on well with us both, and we chat away about her family (Ireland, originally), whether she's married (not yet) and how long she's been nursing. It's really quite sociable.

The ward is pretty quiet, just one or two other patients, all quite a bit older than me, with a relative or friend for company, and Radio 2 is on but not too loudly.

It's a slow process. After a while, though I'm not sure how long, I start to feel sleepy and sick. Emma stops injecting for a moment while we try to work out if it's the cold cap making me feel ill (my head is so cold now I have a headache). I'm not actually sick, though, and after a couple of minutes' break, there's nothing for it but to carry on. My body begins to get cold, and Mark gets me a blanket from another nurse.

Once the first lot of drugs is done, I feel a bit brighter. Drugs two and three are much quicker. The final drug is red in colour, and Emma warns me my pee will turn the same shade as a result. I look at my phone; it's now almost midday and I do some filming.

'Today I'm having my first session of chemotherapy, which is part of my treatment for breast cancer. The chemotherapy drugs are being given to me as a sort of insurance policy – that's how it's been described to me – in case there are any microscopic traces of cancer elsewhere in my body. The chemo will kill them as well as killing all the good cells – ha – but that's the way it goes. On my head I am wearing a cold cap, which is to cool my scalp so it reduces the blood flow, therefore reducing the chemo drugs going to my head, which hopefully should minimise or reduce hair loss, which is one of the side effects of chemo. It may or may not work, but we will see.

'While the drugs were being pushed into me, it felt absolutely all right. What does feel weird is the cap, and the temperature, which is freezing – and that's given me a headache and made me feel sleepy and dozy. I just wanna curl up and go to sleep.

'In the last few days, in the build-up to the chemotherapy, I have been feeling quite vexed and anxious and apprehensive. It's fear of the unknown; of how's it going to affect me, and also I'm really impatient to get the first one under my belt so that I know what I'm dealing with. Right now I've got to wear the cold cap for another hour, so it keeps the scalp cool, but I just feel like I want to go to sleep . . . so I might do just that.'

I give Louisa a quick ring and tell her how it's going. She's incredulous I'm calling her in the middle of it all. I have a notion, I tell her, that if we were still doing our programme on the radio, I might have suggested broadcasting the chemotherapy session live. We discuss whether we really would have done, and what the ethical and practical considerations would have been. On Radio 5 Live we produced and presented a live two-hour broadcast from an abortion clinic in a factual, straightforward way (and didn't receive one complaint afterwards), and did a live broadcast from an animal testing laboratory too. Anyway, it's a wholly theoretical conversation, but it's a welcome diversion, and as always she's full of kindness and encouragement.

My spirits are lifted when all the drugs are in me, but I can't believe I have to keep the cold cap on for another sixty minutes. Emma gives me a red spotted egg-shaped timer so I can make sure I don't do a second longer than I need to. By now I've been wearing it for over two hours, and I feel like my body is beginning to shut down. My eyelids are heavy and I try to sleep, but can't get warm or comfortable. Mark asks for another blanket, and he puts it round my shoulders. Silent tears roll down my face, because having treatment to make you better that first has to make you ill is just miserable. He comforts me and then begins to read to me from the newspaper to try to distract me. I remind myself that I'm wearing this cap to keep my hair, or to keep as much of it as possible, anyway.

At 1 p.m. the bell on the timer rings and it's over. Emma pulls off the cap as I urge her, 'Quick, get it off me!' It's brilliant to be free, and as soon as it's removed, the headache and feelings of nausea vanish. As I touch the top of my head I can feel shards of ice, and Emma points out the ice inside the cap too. Drying my hair with a towel, I feel elated. It's done; we can go. Emma gives me steroids to take each morning for the next couple of days, and also five syringes full of solution I'll have to inject into myself daily from Friday onward, to stimulate the immunity-boosting white blood cells.

Once home, I have a bowl of soup, drink masses of water, because I'm dehydrated, and record some more for my video diary, concluding with this thought: having chemo is like having a vile hangover, which is why I'm glad it's one down, five to go.

As the afternoon wears on I'm increasingly groggy, so go to bed. I can't actually sleep, though; I feel buoyed because I now know what chemotherapy involves, I know what it's like to wear a cold cap and I know what I need to do to cope with it. And by February, this part of the treatment will all be over. Just four months away.

After school, the boys bowl into the bedroom, where I'm dozing. Joe reveals he was sad during maths today and had told his teacher, 'My mum's having chemo and I'm scared.' When I ask Joe what it is that he's frightened of, he says, 'Your brain freezing.' I smile and explain that the cold cap doesn't paralyse your brain, it just makes your head very, very cold.

Before going to sleep (again), I record some more video diary:

'Quick update. It's early evening and I've spent most of the day in bed. As the day has worn on I've felt increasingly queasy and drained. Which is really boring.'

Thursday 5 November

I slept last night but can't get rid of this dull headache. Drinking loads of water to combat dehydration, it still feels as though I'm experiencing an unpleasant, persistent hangover but without any of the fun. I'm lethargic, too, finally getting up (but not dressed) at 4.30 p.m. when the children come back from school. I'm not particularly hungry but eat samosas, with pickle, bizarrely, and a cheese sandwich, also with pickle. I crash out at 8.30 p.m.

Friday 6 November

I wake up at 2.30 a.m. and can't get back to sleep, so get up with the boys at half six. And I feel normal. No headache, no hangover, no lethargy, despite the lack of sleep. The children have porridge for breakfast and I eat loads of fruit, and then I feel fine enough to drive Oliver to the train station and do so, because Mark is like a single dad at the moment, trying to do everything.

I WhatsApp Ben to see if Natalie was like this two days after chemo, adding, 'I could of course relapse at the weekend,' to which he replies, 'I don't ever remember Natalie going backwards with her chemo recovery.'

I take Gracie out for a walk in the light rain, and seeing her haring around, joyful, skittish through the leaves is deeply rewarding. Her happiness makes me happy.

Back home, I set up the camera on my phone and the GoPro at two different angles, to film myself as I prepare to inject drugs into my stomach. I have to build myself up to this because I don't particularly like seeing needles, and normally when one is being stuck into me I simply turn my head. As I'm having to inject myself, I really do have to look at it because I need to see where I'm plunging it in. In the end, with everything treatment-related, the only thing to do is to confront it and get on with it.

I take one of five syringes out of the fridge where they have to be stored, start recording and pull the lid off the needle.

'Woah.' It's so long and vicious-looking, and slavering with solution.

'Sorry, you're going to have to see my belly now,' I say as I grab some flesh on my stomach and with a quick intake of breath, position the needle at an angle, poised to push it into my skin.

I stop there. 'Oh my word, I don't know if I can do this.' Pause. Gather myself. 'OK.' Deep breath.

'Wowww,' I exclaim in a long, low voice, as I gently push the point of the needle into me. It slides in remarkably smoothly. 'The needle's gone in, that's fine, now I've got to push the solution in, push the solution in, all the way in; this is good for me, this is going to boost my immunity, which will protect me from . . . And I've done it! Woo!' I say as I swiftly pull the syringe from my flesh.

I'm a bit shell-shocked. I can't believe I've just done that.

Phew.

Pause.

'OK, that was . . . that was . . . much better than I was expecting.'

It's amazing what you can make yourself do if you have to.

'Oh, the other thing I need to tell you, which is not important but which I'm telling you anyway, is that I haven't washed my hair, or combed my hair, or done anything to my hair, on the advice of nurse Emma, who said the longer you can leave it, then the better it might be for minimising hair loss. So that's why it looks a mess.'

I've been instructed to give myself one of these injections each day for five days, starting forty-eight hours after the chemo session.

Saturday 7 November

Today I'm grumpy (what was my excuse before chemo?).
I feel exhausted, and not as good as I did yesterday, which
seems illogical. Surely as each day goes by you recover some
energy, some strength? The boys and Mark go to watch West
Ham and I take Gracie out, after which I sleep and potter
and mooch around. It's peaceful and relaxing. I brighten up,
and at six-ish drive round to watch *Strictly* and *The X Factor* at
Cathy's and have a takeaway. Paul and their boys and Mark
and our boys join us after their game. By 8.30 p.m. I'm fading
big time, and we leave. I need to get into bed and crash out;
I feel drained. Cathy and Paul completely understand, but I'm
disappointed with myself that I haven't been able to keep up
the pace.

Sunday 8 November

I think I'm going backwards.

Monday 9 November

Am awake between 2 a.m. and 5 a.m. Once I wake up properly, I start to feel reasonably alert. I want to wash my hair but feel apprehensive in case clumps of it fall out. I have to, though; it's so greasy. And no hair falls out. A small triumph. But I have got thrush, due to the steroids. One step forward, two steps back.

I drive into town to get some thrush treatment from Boots and something to help me sleep through the night – just doing that makes me feel a bit more in control. Although by the time I get back I'm so tired again I'm ready for more sleep. I feel flat and discouraged. It's because on Friday, when I was feeling alert, I naively thought I was 'over' the first chemo session. At least I'll be able to manage my expectations next time.

Tuesday 10 November

I slept all the way through last night for the first time in almost a week, having taken the 'night' tablet of 'night and day' tablets.

I can't relax, though, because I can't make a decision about when to go back to work. Outra rings to check up on me and I talk to her about it. She says to bear in mind that with each chemo session it will take longer to recover. That helps me make up my mind – I'm going back on Thursday.

I record a final bit for Video Diary 2.

'It's six days since I've had the first chemotherapy session, and the way it has drained my body has made me feel a bit low. You can feel alert or normal for a couple of hours, and then suddenly this wave of tiredness hits you and you just have to go to bed. That, I have to say, has made me feel a bit disconsolate. As I've said before, everybody reacts differently to treatment, and I hope you don't mind me sharing this with you. There are five more sessions of chemo to go, and this time will pass. And that is something to hold onto.'

Wednesday 11 November

Mark and I watch the video diary of my first chemo session go out on our programme. It feels curious sitting in the warmth of our home observing me experiencing chemo, and makes Mark feel protective towards me, because I look vulnerable on screen and am vulnerable sitting there alongside him, crying. It being on television makes it feel like it's happening to someone else. The film prompts hundreds of messages, including these on Facebook:

> Dear Victoria, I hope this message finds you well and in good spirits despite the challenges of your treatment. As a doctor, I felt compelled to write and tell you how impressed I am by your updates. I cannot begin to emphasise how important your message is to the many people who are about to start treatment for cancer. You have courageously chosen to do something wonderful . . . demystify the reality of treatment. By

allowing people to see what managing cancer really entails, you have helped thousands of patients and family members gain an insight into what is to come. As you so articulately stated, it is often the fear of what is to come that causes such worry. You are doing an amazing job of dispelling the myths of life with cancer. Your honesty and bravery, perceived bad hair day and all (actually you looked great!) are a massive tribute to you. Well done, you're doing something incredible while fighting a hugely personal battle. You should be immensely proud of yourself. There are not many people who can take a terrible situation and turn it into something so positive and helpful for others.

Good luck, stay on the sunny side, sleep well and stand a little taller knowing you are helping others and showing yourself to be hugely brave in the most trying of circumstances.

Best wishes, Dr David Clarke

And this, from a woman recently diagnosed with breast cancer:

Dear Victoria
I would like to thank you from the bottom of my heart. Because you have shared your experience of breast cancer so openly you have made one very scared woman a lot more positive and confident.

I was diagnosed on the day they aired your initial report back in October. I was in the waiting room of the breast clinic waiting to go through to my scan as you came on the television. I'm ashamed to say that at that moment I couldn't deal with watching you and moved away.

Since then I have gone through all the tests, biopsy after biopsy, and all the other stuff that you already know about. Most of the time I have been positive and have said out loud, 'It is what it is and I just have to get on with it.' I'm repeatedly told how brave I am, some have even accused me of being too brave!

The reality is very different: I have been so scared – until now, because I have just watched both your videos and I can't believe how much better I feel. I cried because I felt stronger and happier. That sounds crazy, but I'm sure you'll understand.

All my love and best wishes,

J

These make me feel humbled, and privileged. People are sharing some of their innermost fears with me, because I'm sharing my feelings with them. I feel a deep connection with these strangers – the act of sharing means we're not alone.

And there's this, from the CEO of Macmillan Cancer Support, Lynda Thomas, on Twitter:

Hi @vicderbyshire – just wanted to say I watched your chemo video diary – it's inspiring and helps demystify cancer and its treatments.

In the post is a card from Gloria Hunniford.

Dear Victoria,

You are a VERY SPECIAL GIRL and I admire enormously your TENACITY and STRAIGHTFORWARD ATTITUDE. I really believe the way in which you are dealing with cancer, with all that POSITIVITY, is the way forward. I'm sure you have a few dark days as well, but you are doing a FANTASTIC JOB. I wish you continued STRENGTH and would love to talk with you sometime.

Much love,

Gloria

I feel unutterably grateful for her kind, compassionate words, and unbelievably sad that her daughter isn't here.

Back to work tomorrow, so early bed.

Thursday 12 November

It's a bit like an out-of-body experience reading a newspaper at 4.30 a.m. on my way in to work, and turning over the page to see a picture of me in a cold cap under the headline, 'Honest, raw, brave, inspiring . . . how Britain warmed to BBC Victoria's chemotherapy diary' in the *Daily Mail*. The *Telegraph* says this: 'Derbyshire's film diary to lay bare cancer therapy'. It's as though it's not really me.

It's fabulous being back at work; there's loads to do, no time for much chat but we do have a laugh. Lovely to see everyone in the office after the programme too.

Travelling back home on the train, I begin to fall asleep and on Mark's advice make a decision not to work tomorrow. It's the right thing to do because I sleep for hours when I get home. Maybe I don't have quite as much energy as I want to have.

Friday 13 November

Feeling tired still, but at least normal (although my family should probably be the judge of that).

Anna, one of my closest friends, visits at night and brings me a gift – a piece of art featuring, in the centre, a clock. Around the hands of the clock are the following words: 'There is no such thing as work time; there is no such thing as quality time; there is no such thing as the right time; there is no such thing as downtime; there is no such thing as playtime. There is only time.' It's poignant, and says everything about grabbing life and loving it while you have the opportunity. Over drinks, we spend the evening talking about the recent death of her beloved father, my treatment and life in general.

Tonight, Paris is attacked by terrorists.

Monday 16 November

I go to work, I come home, Mark makes a cottage pie, we eat together as a family. It's special because it's so normal.

Tuesday 17 November

A survivor of the Paris terrorist attack, Thomas Tran Dinh, speaks eloquently on our programme about hate and love. We introduce him to a survivor of the 7/7 bombings, of the Mumbai shootings and the Tunisia beach attack. I listen as they converse together and share their experiences. Our audience tells us it's powerful and moving. It's a reminder of how strong some people can be in the face of adversity.

Wednesday 18 November

On air, we cover the unfolding hunt for the Paris terrorists as police target a suburb of the French capital. One female suspect blows herself up with a suicide vest and another suspect is shot dead.

After the programme, Louisa and I go to meet Shaker Aamer, a British resident released just over two weeks ago from the US military prison at Guantanamo Bay. I'm interviewing him soon, as are ITN, and this is where we sound him out and he sounds us out.

His last child was born on the day he was taken to the prison in Cuba – Valentine's Day 2001. Since we've worked at Radio 5 Live, Louisa and I have regularly reported on his continued detention without trial after being arrested by American soldiers in Afghanistan during the so-called 'war on terror'. He's not what I am expecting. Considering his years locked up, physically he looks extremely well. Mentally, I have no idea. He smiles and says he's not angry or bitter at what has happened to him. His voice is booming and commanding and he talks a lot – but then he has a lot to say. Going to be interesting interviewing him when we fix a date.

Saturday 21 November

It's Paul's fortieth birthday party. Back in the summer, after I was diagnosed, making sure I was at this event was one of my priorities. My aim was to have treatment done and dusted by today. How naive I was in the early days of cancer. But at least I'm here, along with all of Paul's close friends and family, in a Surrey hotel preparing to celebrate.

As I wash my hair over the bath, several long, wet strands suddenly begin to collect in the plughole. Not loads, but enough for me to know that this is down to the chemo.

It's a surprise, but I'm unruffled, and as I see some of the hair detaching itself from my head, I say out loud, 'Oh, wow.'

'What is it, darlin'?' Mark calls from the bedroom.

'My hair's falling out,' I say in a deadpan voice.

In the seventeen days that have passed since I wore the cold cap, I've been secretly thinking I'd got away with it; I was the one for whom the cold cap would work 100 per cent.

As I start to dry it with the hairdryer, a little more comes out, this time in a clump. I'm pretty cheery, considering – I'm about to attend a big celebration, after all – and film a bit for my third video diary, which will inevitably be called 'Hair Loss'.

'I'm in a hotel room and I'm getting ready to go to a friend's fortieth downstairs. It's two and a half weeks since the first chemo session and it's four days until the second . . . and I just wanted to show you this [holding up a fistful of dry hair in my hand]. This is the first bit of hair that has fallen out. I was prepared for it . . . obviously it's a side effect of chemotherapy, but it's slightly disconcerting nevertheless.'

I dress, and Mark and I go downstairs, where we have the best night with all of Paul and Cathy's fabulous friends. I feel proud of staying up till 3 a.m. It's a bit lightweight, though – most of the others party for another couple of hours.

Monday 23 November

Two days before chemotherapy, I go to the hospital to have a chat with the oncologist, who checks how I'm doing, and to have a blood test to ensure that my white blood cell count is back to normal. If it isn't, chemo will have to be delayed. Dr Teoh asks if I've had any sickness – I haven't, presumably because of the steroids I've taken in the run-up to and immediately after chemo. I feel well, but I am definitely becoming anxious about more hair falling out, but there's little Dr Teoh can do about the fact that I keep finding strands around the house.

A beautiful candle and card arrive from Shelagh – 'A little light for the chemo phase,' she writes. She is so thoughtful.

Wednesday 25 November

Chemo session 2: I drop Ollie at the train station and Joe off at Cathy's. She's taking him to school because Mark and I need to be at the hospital for 9 a.m. This time I take my own blankets because I know how cold it's going to be. I'm sanguine about the next couple of hours – I've got one under my belt – but less so about the prospect of further drugs leading to more hair loss. 'To plant the seed in your head', as she puts it, nurse Emma suggests shaving all my hair off to avoid the stress of seeing bits of it gradually fall out over the coming weeks.

'No way.' I'm emphatic. It's impossible for me even to imagine taking clippers to my hair and shaving it – it would be too grimly distressing.

I'm happy to see a new modern-looking cold cap (pink, inevitably) with a more sophisticated cooling machine which has recently been delivered by Paxman (not him, but the company that manufactures them). It fits much more snugly, and, crucially, can be placed on my head at room temperature and cooled once in place, which means I can avoid the vicious freeze from the moment it goes on. Plus I'm able to take paracetamol this time, so that should prevent a headache. That wasn't allowed three weeks ago, as the painkillers could have masked any adverse reaction to the chemo drugs.

The infusion itself is absolutely fine: there are no problems, no feelings of nausea. I'm wrapped up in my soft grey blanket and manage to watch our programme on the iPad. More contemporary this new cold cap may be, but once the drugs are administered, Emma says I need to wear it for another *ninety* minutes. That's almost inhumane. I set the red egg timer again. Outra pops in to say hi, which distracts me for a while. And then I film a bit more.

'Hello! It's Wednesday the twenty-fifth of November, and I've just finished my second chemotherapy session, and it has felt much better this time. I'm wearing a different cold cap – apparently it's a new generation of cold cap: it's closer-fitting, and has a much more efficient cooling system. And you can probably see on there [pointing at the machine] I've got forty-eight minutes to go. So after the drugs have gone into me, I have to wear it for another hour . . . no, another hour and a half, I beg your pardon, to keep the scalp cool, hopefully to minimise hair loss. A bit of hair has been coming out, but not that much at this stage. I haven't had a bad headache like I had last time. Perhaps it's just because I'm more used to it, or I know what to expect. But I would say, compared to last time, it's fifty per cent better. I've been much more alert, not half as sleepy, and, um, just a bit more cheerful, really.'

The timer goes, and as Emma takes off the cap we film the ice on top of my head and inside the cap.

I spend most of the rest of the day in bed. When I wake, I need water.

Friday 27 November

It's incredible how much I'm sleeping. Last night I turned the light off at 10 p.m. and slept until 3.45 a.m. Eventually I dozed off again until 8 a.m., and I need to go back and get more sleep at 11 a.m. for a couple of hours. 'Listen to your body,' everyone says, so I am. Imagine doing twelve rounds in a boxing match before running a marathon – that's about how knackered I am.

This afternoon I try to wash my hair. A simple, mundane task becomes a nightmare. When I start to rub shampoo in, it begins to get matted. The more it mats, the more hassled yet determined I become to de-mat it. As I lean over the bath, I can see long hairs slipping from my head into the plughole, while the rest of the hair continues to tangle and twist together on my head. When I stare into the bathroom mirror, I look like Mr Rochester's wild wife from *Jane Eyre* – hair sticking up, out, uncontrollable. I wrap a towel round my head and consider how much hair is falling out after just two chemo cycles, while wearing the cold cap. It's depressing. Then, a positive to counterbalance the negative – but if I hadn't worn the cap, it could have been worse.

I put on a beanie hat to hide the lot and set off for an appointment with Amy to collect my wig, which is ready. Good timing.

By the time I get to her salon, I'm pretty stressed as I reveal the mess on my head. She doesn't bat an eyelid. Her pragmatic yet kind manner is reassuring. She's seen it all before, and explains what's happening: the hair that's falling out has got caught in the hair that remains on my head – hence a tangled shambles. She sits me down in front of her mirror and begins carefully to brush it out. It takes a good twenty minutes to comb through the knots, leaving a large clump of it on her floor. As I watch, tears balance in my eyes but don't spill over onto my cheeks.

Then she brings in my handmade wig on the mannequin head. I'm taken aback by how much like my hair it is – the colour, the cut, the length, the style. I'm quietly thrilled – this is the one thing that's going to help me carry on working over the next few months. My emotions are so volatile – one moment in tears, the next elated. Amy demonstrates how to put it on.

I clip what's left of my hair to my head, making a smooth base. Then, holding the front of the wig with both my thumb and forefinger on each hand, I hold it above my head and slip it onto the forehead first, before gently pulling it backward at the base of the wig so it fits properly. It feels snug. Next, I take some double-sided sticky tape, already cut into strips for exactly this purpose, and stick one on my skin next to each ear, before pushing the lace cap of the wig onto it. It's definitely fiddly, but Amy says the more I do it, the easier and quicker it will become.

Then I stare at myself in the mirror. I'm me, but with a wig on – a wig that looks remarkably like my own hair, yet to me it's clearly not my own hair. I say nothing, and nor does Amy. It takes a few seconds to absorb the way it looks. In my head there's disbelief that I'm in a situation which means I need to wear a wig. But it looks . . . sort of all right.

Finally and tentatively I say, 'OK . . . it looks . . . OK. Doesn't it? Or does it not?' I'm so unsure because it's crazy even to be wearing a wig at all. Yet it does look remarkably like my real hair. I smile unexpectedly, which leads Amy to do the same. She's done a pretty incredible job. I sit there for a few minutes just looking at my 'new' self in the mirror.

And then I want to take it off. As I remove it, I express anxiety about how secure it is, and whether it will blow off in strong wind, for example, but Amy says in her many years' experience, definitely not. I ask if I can take home the hair that's fallen out.

'Are you sure you want to?' she asks.

I am.

I drive home feeling troubled. Alan arrives to trim my real hair, and to cut a few more layers in the wig.

'Alan, I might cry as I explain all this, but my hair is now coming out, so can you cut the wig, please, into my usual style and just trim around what's left of my real hair?'

'Don't worry, of course. We can do whatever we need to; please don't worry.'

As I take the wig out of the box and place it on the mannequin head, he is amazed at how real it looks, describing it as 'fab', which gives me a boost, to be honest. He cuts my real hair into a very short bob. As so much has fallen out or been brushed out today, it's very thin on top, particularly at the front. About half of my hair remains. Losing my hair bothers me much, much more than losing a breast. Why is that? Because without your hair, you don't look like you.

Having attached the wig, Alan trims it so it looks similar to how my hair used to be. He does a brilliant job, but I cannot process this at all. It feels absolutely brutal. Once it's cut, I place it back on the mannequin; I don't want to wear it in the house in case I mess it up.

Despite my real hair now being in a new flapper-girl-type meagre bob, the boys and Mark still see me as normal. Yet I'm distressed, and feel like hiding.

Saturday 28 November

The morning's spent worrying about my hair, debating whether I feel strong enough, physically and mentally, to go to Richard Bacon's fortieth tonight, and also working – reading through briefs on Shaker Aamer and considering what questions I'll put to him. We don't have a date fixed for the interview yet, but I'm fretful it will be too near the next chemo session for me to be alert enough.

Cathy pops round at lunchtime, and I'm upstairs reading. I can hear her chatting to Mark, and it occurs to me to stay in the bedroom and hide myself and my 'new' thin, short hair, but in the end I force myself to go down to the kitchen. She doesn't react when she sees me (apart from saying hi), as I apologise for my appearance.

'Sorry, Cathy, I'm not intending to frighten you to death, but that may happen.'

She smiles.

'Well, what's my excuse then? My hair's like that without chemo!' It makes me laugh.

Later, I put my make-up on and practise attaching my wig to see

a) if I can do it
b) how I look.

I know I'm trying to work out if I feel confident enough to go to Richard's party. I don't think I do, and I'm deflated but call him in a cheery voice to apologise.

This is shit.

Sunday 29 November

On the phone to my brother Nick, I tell him how low I'm feeling because my hair's falling out. I cry the most I've cried since the day I was diagnosed at the end of July. He attempts to comfort me, but it's hard because there's little he can say apart from a gentle reminder that the chemo might protect me against the cancer coming back in the future.

'Might protect me. Might! You go through all this, and there's not even a hundred per cent guarantee that it won't come back,' I say resentfully.

I'm a rational person: I like making decisions based on evidence, and I love facts. Therefore I know my hair will grow back. And yet there is something in my brain that's making me think, what if it doesn't come back? Or it grows back white? (it happens occasionally, apparently); or it grows back and it's not as thick and shiny as it once was? The sensible bit of my brain is fighting with the irrational bit, which is contaminated by doubts and fears caused by this illness.

Monday 30 November

I'm low, vexed and distressed. I know I'm losing my positivity.

I record some more for my video diary, wearing my wig, which no one knows about:

'It's now six days since the second chemotherapy session, and like the first one, I'm at the stage where I'm feeling dispirited. One of the things I'm finding it difficult to come to terms with is losing my hair. I would say I have lost about thirty to fifty per cent of my hair.'

Then I remove my wig directly in front of the camera to reveal my shorter, thinning hair.

'And I'm finding this hard,' I say, with tears in my eyes.

I pick Joe up from school wearing the beanie hat, not the wig. As he climbs into the car he turns to me and says, 'You look nice today.'

Tuesday 1 December

I make two decisions, both of which help me regain some control, having lost all control of what happens with my hair: I'm going back to work tomorrow, and I'm going to wear the wig properly for the first time.

I'm edgy and agitated, though, so practise putting it on and sticking it down a couple of times. I'm forcing myself to go back tomorrow, because the sooner I get on with wearing it, the more normal it will become for me. Physically I feel fine; mentally I know it's about confronting my anxiety over wearing a wig in front of friends, colleagues and our TV audience.

Wednesday 2 December

I'm awake for a couple of hours in the night before the alarm goes off at 3.30 a.m. – I've set it even earlier to give me time to put my wig on carefully. It feels like a huge hurdle for me today.

Louisa knows, of course, and she's promised to tell me on talkback (from where she sits in the TV gallery, through my earpiece) if the wig moves or looks peculiar or bizarre at any point throughout our two-hour programme. That's my biggest worry. Carol, one of our lovely make-up artists, knows too. I'm somewhat paranoid about being on television and viewers realising because it looks obvious or unnatural; and I'm not ready to tell everyone yet because I want to get used to wearing it myself first. Just before I go on air at 9 a.m., Carol comes into the studio to do a final make-up/hair check. Under my breath, so none of the cameramen and -women can hear, I say, 'Can you tell?' She beckons me to the side of the studio away from everyone and just gives it a slight tug forward on my head, before saying, 'No, not now!' We can't help giggling conspiratorially. It's farcical.

As soon as the programme starts I forget about my appearance. As always, I'm totally engaged in the stories. It's a big news day – MPs are debating whether Britain should take part in air strikes in Syria and the programme is incredibly busy, with plenty of interviews for me to focus on. It's a joy simply to get on with the job.

When it's over, the tension in my body dissipates – it's a relief to get one show under my belt while wearing a wig. Mark, Cathy and Juliet all text to say it looks good and that no one could tell. I record a bit for my video diary in the make-up room after the programme:

'It's a week after the second chemo session, and I've gone to work. It's brilliant to see everybody, and be back in the routine and work with people on the programme again; and I feel normal. And that's good – feeling normal is good.'

Later I realise I've gone back to work a day earlier than I did after the first chemo cycle. It feels like a minor triumph.

Outside the school gates, a couple of the mums I don't know too well ask me how I'm doing and offer to help in any way they can, either by picking Joe up or coming round to make me a sandwich for lunch. I've met more good women in the last few months that in most of the rest of my life.

Friday 4 December

Leaving the studios after work, I feel tired but also a sense of achievement for having worked three days this week. Three! In a row! And wearing a wig, with hopefully very few people realising (apart from my mum and sister, who will have known as soon as they saw me on TV in it, although we haven't talked about it yet).

Saturday 5 December

It's Joe's ninth birthday. I wake at 6.30 a.m. and the boys come into our bedroom at 8 a.m. for cards and gifts. Both are in a brilliant mood, and Joe is totally delighted with his shiny new white iPod. I'm totally delighted too, to be here witnessing my younger son celebrate his birthday.

Sunday 6 December

Mark takes the children to their respective football matches while I spend several more hours reading up on Shaker Aamer ahead of the interview, which is now scheduled for tomorrow. ITN too have secured an interview with him, and we will be allowed to release both broadcasts at exactly the same time. The arrangements are that both teams will arrive first thing, we will each have two hours with him – not a minute more – and we'll use the same camera people to avoid wasting time setting up new cameras and lights in between. Mr Aamer's lawyers are treating us, quite rightly, equally. Louisa asked ITN last week if we could go first, because I get tired the longer the day goes on. They said no and suggested, instead, tossing a coin – we lost.

It's Joe's party in the afternoon, and lots of boys start arriving from 3 p.m onward.

Monday 7 December

I've done so much preparation for the interview with Shaker Aamer, I feel alert and OK. We arrive at a firm of solicitors in London at 9 a.m. and hang around for hours waiting for ITN to complete their filming with him. Mr Aamer's hair is tied neatly into a low ponytail and he's wearing a pale blue shirt, chinos and black trainers. Finally we start at about 1 p.m. I ask him about arriving back on British soil, and insight into what it's like seeing his wife and children for the first time in nearly fourteen years, including his youngest child, who he's never met; why he moved to Kabul with his family in 2001, ruled by the Taliban; how he knows a British intelligence officer was present when he was being tortured, having been captured by the Americans after 9/11. Then I say this:

Me: I'd like to read to you a list of claims
made against you — all of which come from an
official US Department of Defense file from
November 2007, which concluded that you were
high-risk, that you were likely to pose a
threat to the US, its interests and its
allies.

SA: None of the allegations is true, what
they've been saying about me.

At this point Mr Aamer's lawyer interrupts to object. We explain
that it's important for the questions to be put to him in order
for him to be able to respond. If we don't ask the questions, the
audience won't have the opportunity to hear his answers. The
lawyer's doing her job, I suppose, although Shaker Aamer himself seems content to answer whatever I ask.

I begin again.

Me: You were an Al Qaeda operative, they said.

SA: Not at all. Prove it. Prove it. Prove
anything that you say is true — prove it. Prove
it to the world.

Me: You held a senior position in a UK-based Al
Qaeda cell.

SA: Again, allegations.

Me: You're a close associate of Osama bin
Laden.

SA: Keep going . . . when? How? Where is the
evidence? Where is the British intelligence at
that time? Five years I'd been living in this
country; how come I was an operative for bin
Laden, working in London, and they didn't even
know about it?

Me: You never communicated with him?

SA: Not at all.

Me: You never met him?

SA: Definitely not . . . and if the British
say otherwise, why didn't you give it to the
Americans to prove that I was communicating
with him?

I can hear the lawyer sitting in the corner of the room, whispering loudly and furiously to Louisa in tones that suggest she's very unhappy with the line of questioning. I keep going.

Me: Another accusation — you were an Al Qaeda
recruiter, financier and facilitator, with a
history of participating in jihadist combat.

SA: Definitely not . . . it's a joke.

Me: The file goes on to say that you had links
to well-known jihadists such as the Jordanian
cleric Abu Qatada, like Abu Hamza, former imam
at the Finsbury Park Mosque in London.

SA: I do know Abu Hamza, truly . . . and I will be lying if I say I *know* him. I know *of* him, because he was in the mosque. Abu Qatada used to pray in his place, I used to sit and listen to his speeches, and I know he's not a bad guy. That's exactly what I know; I know he's not a bad guy, and he's not somebody horrible, as they say he is.

Me: Described by a Spanish judge as 'Osama bin Laden's right-hand man in Europe' . . .

SA: I don't know about that, but according to my own knowledge, he's got nothing to do with bin Laden, and he never preached about him in his circle, and he never encouraged anybody to go to Afghanistan.

Me: And one final one from that Department of Defense file: you admitted, it says, that you associated with the convicted shoe bomber Richard Reid.

SA: Lies.

Me: This file, containing all those accusations against you, came out in November 2007, several months after you'd been cleared for release by the Bush administration.

SA: Amazing, isn't it?

Me: So what do you think was going on?

```
SA: It's amazing; I'll just leave the audience
to think about it. I mean, these allegations
came out after they cleared me. And yet, after
they cleared me they found all that out?
```

Mr Aamer goes on to describe how, on being transferred to the American detention facility at Guantanamo Bay on the Caribbean island of Cuba, US guards tried to 'break him', both physically and psychologically. He talks about being forced onto the cold floor as his arms were handcuffed behind him and then shackled to his legs; how, he says, he was kept in isolation for two years and ten months and made 'friends' with ants in his cell; how he helped look after a stray cat whom he named Amira, to give him some purpose during solitary confinement; that he read *Harry Potter and the Prisoner of Azkaban* and editions of *Good Housekeeping* magazine. He also tells us he always knew he would get out because 'I know I did not do *anything* wrong, and I know justice will prevail.'

We get twenty minutes less than ITN in the end because the lawyer decides we've asked enough. I think everyone feels drained by this stage, including Mr Aamer, because it's been pretty full on.

Tuesday 8 December

Work. Love work.

Thursday 10 December

Today I'm being 'inducted' into what's called the Radio Academy Hall of Fame. The boys think it's an actual building, inside which is a gallery containing the portraits of famous radio names: Annie Nightingale, Chris Evans, John Humphrys.

What it means is travelling to Birmingham for a lunch, after which people make speeches about you before you say a few words. Mark decides the boys should come and witness this, and their respective schools are happy to give permission (if I hadn't had cancer, would we have taken the boys? Probably not. The diagnosis means these kinds of events take on a greater intensity). Also being awarded a place in the 'hall' today are Frank Skinner, Nihal Arthanayake, Pete Tong and Tony Butler, who's worked in radio in the Midlands for decades.

I feel self-conscious about wearing a wig. The boys reassure me no one will notice and, of course, no one seems to, or if they do, they certainly don't say anything. I'm irritated that I'm feeling so vexed – for God's sake, I've been on television wearing it, what's the problem? It's because I'll be up close with people I've known for years, and if anyone's going to spot it, it's them. The boys look at me no differently with the wig on, or with my gradually thinning hair. I tell them my hair looks not unlike the West Ham manager's, Slaven Bilić, which they love.

We nearly miss the train from Euston, which Louisa is sitting on patiently. Running from the tube to the train, the wig stays secure – a good omen.

It is a truly special afternoon – some of our wonderful friends from Radio 5 Live are here – Sophie, Jane and Jonny; Elaine and Monica who now work on our TV programme, as well as my old boss, Ceri Thomas, who, in a speech to introduce me onto the stage, says some unbelievably gorgeous things about the way I've done my job over the years. Then it's my turn. I'm incredibly nervous, for all sorts of reasons – I'm wearing a wig, I'm having treatment for cancer, I'm not as strong as I usually am, the audience is a room full of my radio peers, my sons and partner are watching, plus I've had a glass and a half of wine and hardly eaten any lunch. My voice wavers to begin with, and then I get into a rhythm and settle down. I thank so many people: Ceri, a brilliant editor, the first editor who actually gave me the confidence to think I could interview anyone; Louisa, bold and brave editorially; Bob Shennan, who gave me the opportunity to present my own programme on Radio 5 Live when he was the controller; the radio community – colleagues and listeners – for being so supportive when I was diagnosed, and end by telling everyone that Mark and I have definitely passed our love of radio down to our boys. They adore Capital, 5 Live Sport, Radio 2 and *Just a Minute* on Radio 4.

Monday 14 December

We put the whole interview with Shaker Aamer up on YouTube today, all ninety-three minutes of it; and on our programme broadcast it in three parts, lasting around fifteen minutes each. While it's going out, I'm having a blood test to see if my white cell count has recovered enough to have chemo on Wednesday. I travel into work afterwards to voice up a report about Aamer for the 1 p.m. TV bulletin, which also goes out later on the BBC's ten o'clock news.

Tuesday 15 December

A cancer charity called Maggie's has asked if I'll host a podcast for them to mark World Cancer Day in February, and I have my first meeting with the executive producer, Maria Williams. She's a tour de force; we swap ideas, and I can't wait to do some radio again. As always, scheduling in the recording of the podcast fits in around chemo and the time it takes to recover from each session.

Louisa and I then meet Dan Wootton, the showbiz editor of the *Sun*, for a fabulously gossipy lunch.

I receive a Christmas card, sent to the office, from David and Samantha Cameron. This has never happened before, so conclude it must be because I have cancer. In reality it simply means I've somehow got onto a Downing Street press officer's list somewhere, yet I can't help but feel touched.

Wednesday 16 December

Cathy texts to say good luck, as she always does, it seems, whenever I have an appointment at the hospital. I don't know how she remembers every time, especially as she's one of the busiest women I know – two kids, full-time job, manager of one of the local junior football teams *and* she's doing a PhD.

It's the third cycle of chemotherapy – halfway through – *yes*. I take in champagne and chocolates to give all the staff for Christmas. I'm so blasé about today's session; Mark goes to watch Joe's Christmas assembly at school before joining me mid-morning with a cheese sandwich and water. Emma starts off administering the drugs, but then her colleague in the Infusion Suite, Sue, takes over. It never ceases to amaze me how much you can learn about an individual's life in an hour or so while they're injecting drugs into you. Sue's good company, and fills me in about her husband, children and grandchildren.

I record my video diary of the session.

'Hello again, it's December the sixteenth, and today is a small milestone in the course of this chemotherapy treatment because I've just finished the third one, which means I'm halfway through, and that's quite a satisfying feeling. The time is passing quickly, which surprises me; and if you are experiencing this, or someone you know is experiencing this treatment, then keep on keeping on because it will pass.'

I sleep most of the afternoon and wake to lovely texts from my mum, Alex and Nick.

Friday 18 December

At half seven, I eat breakfast, take an anti-sickness tablet and go straight back to bed. It's our work Christmas lunch today, and I'm determined to go. I love our team, and don't want to miss our first-ever festive party. I recall this time last year as we were preparing to launch our programme; there were five of us for Christmas dinner – Monica, a senior journalist on the programme, Harriet, our assistant editor, Jim, our reporter, Louisa and me. It was very special, and we had a real laugh, but today's will be even better. Mark wonders aloud about the wisdom of me travelling into central London on public transport when my immunity is so low, but I tell him I honestly don't think it will be a problem (even if it is, I'm determined to go).

I wake up again at 11 a.m. and get ready. Sitting at my dressing table, putting mascara and lipstick on, I feel spaced out, slightly dizzy and every movement I make appears to be in slow motion. Concentrating as I look in the mirror, I pull my wig on, a task that becomes easier and quicker each time I do it.

Before leaving I inject into my stomach the solution that boosts my immune system, thinking I might need it more than usual once I'm on the train surrounded by other people and their winter germs.

Louisa meets me off the tube and I'm so hungry we pop into a mini-supermarket for a sandwich on the walk to the restaurant. There's a huge turnout – producers, reporters, cameramen and -women, sound technicians and Barry our talented director, and we all sit at a great long trestle table and in booths around the sides of the room. Although I like the notion of a beer or glass of wine, in reality I can't face it and drink water. It feels wonderful to be there and not missing out, knowing I'd be resentful if I hadn't managed to make it. Elaine and Sarah H. on our team present some daft and clever programme awards – including producers Adam and Sarah B. winning a trophy for 'best double act' (they turn up for work inadvertently wearing matching outfits – and they are not a couple); an award for Claire, one of our senior journalists, for being super-chirpy 100 per cent of the time; and a prize for Jim for staying all hours of the night to create perfect reports before they go out on air. It's a lively, fun afternoon, but by five I'm done and I have to get home. Saying goodbye seems to take a long time, and I feel slightly anxious about travelling back in rush hour and so want to get on with it. It's absolutely fine; just hot on the packed train. Once I collect the boys from their friends and we reach home, I feel secure. Finally I relax and start looking forward to Christmas.

Sunday 20 December

I've had enough of chemotherapy now. The routine of spending days sleeping, eating, drinking water and then sleeping again is interrupting my life. I hate feeling weak and under strength. I want this to be behind me. The third session is definitely taking longer to bounce back from – it must be the cumulative effect of the drugs that Outra warned me about.

When I allow myself for a split second to think of the future, I feel optimistic. I imagine being completely cancer-free, of not thinking about cancer or talking about it, of doing all the things we normally do but without the shadow of this brutal treatment hanging over me.

At night we go to Cathy's for Christmas drinks. As we're getting ready, Oliver says, 'It doesn't matter to me what your hair looks like, or whether you wear a wig or not, it's what kind of person you are inside.' My heart almost bursts. Through this treatment my boys have had a habit of saying exactly the right things. I love them deeply and am so proud of them.

It's a lovely evening with plenty of laughs. When we get back, Joe tells me in a protective way that no one would have known I was wearing a wig.

Monday 21 December

Oliver's got a job as a paper boy, and he's thrilled.

Tuesday 22 December

Mark takes the boys to work because they love going into Radio 2 with him. It's miserable and blowy outside, but in my warm kitchen, sitting on the floor in my dressing gown with Gracie on my lap, listening to Chris Evans's infectious, happy tones on his breakfast show, I feel buoyant. As a broadcaster he makes me feel upbeat in normal times, but when you're feeling more flat than usual, his lively outlook lifts me. The Lewisham and Greenwich NHS Choir are guests on his programme this morning and they sing 'A Bridge Over You' – their stunning mash-up of Simon and Garfunkel's 'Bridge Over Troubled Water', and Coldplay's 'Fix You'. I get emotional listening to them because

a) it's beautiful
b) it's a choir made up of NHS staff
c) it's nearly Christmas.

Eating breakfast, I realise that as well as a medium-sized mouth ulcer, which is slightly painful, I have a constant taste of thick paper in my mouth – more side effects – hurray! Neither is a big deal, though. I put my wig on as Anna's coming round to drop off some Christmas presents for the boys. She doesn't know I've been wearing it on TV, and when I tell her she is genuinely surprised and says that not for a second would she ever have guessed. To be honest, it's a relief to reveal it. I'm not enjoying having this secret. I know why I've kept it hidden – because I need to get used to wearing it before I let anyone else know. But like all secrets, this one too is becoming a burden. It's dull wasting time wondering if people are looking at you differently because they're trying to work out if you're wearing a wig, when in reality I know they're probably not. Not since getting ready to go out on a Friday night as a teenager have I ever spent so much brainpower worrying about my appearance, and it's tedious.

When Oliver, Joe and Mark arrive home from a day at the

office, the boys can't *wait* to tell me that they met Chris Evans today. They are full of it: how charming he was, how they went into his studio while the choir were there, how cramped it was with around twenty people in a confined space, how he let them press the button to fire some jingles, had a photo with them – all while he was doing his job. I would love it if an experience like today inspires them to go into radio when they're older.

Drive round to make-up lady Carol's house in the evening and leave a bottle of champagne on her doorstep to thank her for her extraordinary kindness towards me over the last few months.

So tired by 8 p.m. I go to bed.

Thursday 24 December

Physically I'm finally feeling back to normal, which cheers me greatly, just in time for tomorrow, and record another update next to the decorated tree as Gracie wriggles around on my lap:

'It's Christmas Eve, and it's taken me eight days to bounce back from the last session of chemotherapy. I've spent a week doing a lot of sleeping and feeling a bit dizzy, and having this disgusting cardboard taste in my mouth; I've had one mouth ulcer, but only one, so it's not the end of the world. Also, I have got used to wearing a wig, which is something I never thought I would be able to say. The idea, a few weeks ago, of wearing a wig absolutely horrified me. It represented stress, it represented something peculiar, and was not me, and now I can put it on in five minutes in the morning . . . it lets me crack on and just get on with things, which is absolutely great.'

Friday 25 December

We all pile down to my brother's house in Wiltshire, and enjoy one of the best Christmases ever. Nick, his wife Katie and their little boy, my nephew, have pulled out all the stops to make it extra special. Although it's unspoken, there's a significant undercurrent among us that life really can be cut short, so we have to make the most of these times when we're all together – us three siblings, our partners, our children and our mum.

We drink, chat and laugh while Nick and Katie prepare the food; I talk to my sister and Mum for the first time about my wig – they both knew immediately, of course, when they saw me in it on TV. Secretly I was hoping it was so good even they wouldn't spot it, but of course they did – they're the two women who know me best.

Sitting down to lunch, I reflect on being here and reaching this milestone – Christmas Day – right in the middle of my chemotherapy treatment. Soon a brand-new year will begin, which means soon treatment will be over. I can't wait for cancer to be behind me.

After lunch, Nick makes a beautiful speech featuring every one of us, including all the children, referencing our individual challenges, foibles, achievements and hopes for 2016. It's both moving and funny, as we heckle at various points throughout.

Sunday 27 December

I don't want to leave. Being together like this is such fun.

Monday 28 December

Louisa sends me a link to a *Sunday Telegraph* article from yesterday of the 'Fifty Greatest Britons 2015'. I click on it on my phone and start to scroll through it – David Cameron, Nicola Sturgeon, Jeremy Corbyn, Adele – and suddenly my name is there, in black and white, at Number Two, JUST BEHIND THE BLOODY QUEEN!! This is absurd. 'Oh my God,' I say to Mark and the boys as I read the piece. Adele, smart, talented, funny, normal, amazing Adele – I'm above Adele!! It's ridiculous, and also flattering . . .

> *In a bravura piece of reporting, BBC journalist Victoria Derbyshire – talking direct to camera from an NHS hospital bed hours after having breast cancer surgery in October [it was September, but hey] – stunned and impressed us all with her raw honesty. Her defiant display of courage, designed to offer hope to the 58,000 Britons who are diagnosed with this disease every year, began with Derbyshire, 46, holding up a handwritten sign saying: 'This morning I had breast cancer'. And then another sign saying, 'This evening I don't!' Derbyshire was documenting her illness via a video diary in order to demystify*

the experience for others. She is now undergoing chemotherapy and sharing that treatment with viewers, while she continues to work.

It puts an extra spring in my step.

Tuesday 29 December

My mood is ... brilliant. I feel well, and for the first time in months, totally relaxed. I haven't felt like this since the last time I was on leave and didn't know I had cancer, although I now realise the mutating cells were there then, lurking sinisterly inside me. That was June.

Video diary:

'It's the end of the year, and like you, no doubt, I'm looking forward to the year ahead. I cannot WAIT for 2016 to get cracking, I really can't, particularly the last few days of February when chemotherapy will end. Hurray. Then I'll have a little bit of radiotherapy, but everybody who's had radiotherapy says that compared to chemo, it's an absolute breeze. Quick health update: I have another ulcer; I have a little bit of brown mottling on my face; I've lost a little of my eyebrows, but you just fill in the missing bits with an eyebrow pencil. I have managed to preserve my nails, perhaps because I received some advice that said if you wear dark nail varnish it helps to maintain them through chemo, so that appears to be working, which is good.

I cannot wait to get back to work, albeit briefly, before the next session of chemo starts. When I started wearing a wig a few weeks ago I didn't tell anyone at work that I was wearing one because I needed a little time to adjust to it myself. I can confirm that I am now fully adjusted to it, so I feel comfortable in being totally open about it. But we are a close-knit team at work, and they are a bunch of journalists, so I'm guessing they've sussed it already, and if they haven't, I'll be a bit disappointed, to be honest!

'During the course of treatment, the side effect of losing my hair has been the distressing part for me. It has been the thing that has affected me the most, more than a mastectomy, which may sound peculiar, but maybe not. As I've said before, everybody's different, but that's certainly the way I have felt about it.

'But hey, my hair will grow back. So that's cool. And . . . roll on 2016! I hope you have a brilliant year ahead, and thank you, thank you, thank you for your thoughtful and kind and inspiring messages – they have meant such a lot to me.'

Thursday 31 December

I wash and blow-dry my wig. It takes ages – two hours of my life I won't get back. Using wig pins, I secure it to the polystyrene head it sits on before placing that in the bath. Using the shower attachment, I wet the hair all over and then gently smooth shampoo on it, from the top to the ends, before rinsing and applying conditioner.

The time-consuming bit is the blow-drying, because there is so much hair. I put a few Velcro rollers in to give it some body and leave it for several hours in our bedroom. It's made Mark jump a few times when he walks in at night and sees the silhouette of what appears to be a severed head with flowing hair casually sitting on my dressing table.

In the evening, Mark, the boys and I go to the panto at Richmond Theatre (*Cinderella*), which is fun and Christmassy and daft because Matthew Kelly and Hayley Mills are very entertaining, and then on to Wagamama's. I love spending this time with Oliver and Joe; they are such good company. Once we get back, we all sit round the island in the kitchen with champagne, the boys with hot milk, chatting and laughing and talking about what we might do in the coming year . . .

1. Throw a summer 'thank you' party for all the friends and family who've been so considerate to us in the last few months
2. Go to Northumberland for a fix of North-East sky, sea and beaches
3. Fundraise for our local hospital – Mark's into doing a sponsored bike ride, and the boys say they would like to do a 2K or 3K run.

The conversation is upbeat and life-affirming. The boys beg to stay up till midnight, but by about half ten they are tired and upstairs they go.

When midnight strikes, Mark and I hold each other securely. I shed tears of relief that 2015 is ending.

Friday 1 January 2016

I adore this feeling only a new year can bring. Optimism, a clean slate, everything being possible. I feel well and happy and exchange upbeat texts with Elaine, Helena, Laurence, Anna and Louisa. Potter around the house, tidy the boys' bedrooms and then relax with *Homes & Gardens* magazine and a book on antiques that Mark's bought me. Bliss.

Sunday 3 January

Oliver started his new job yesterday – a paper round – and Mark and Gracie went with him, just to check he was safe. Today I want to keep him company, so we're up at 7 a.m. It's cold and misty, and Gracie loves being out first thing investigating the leftover scent of night-time foxes. The route takes about half an hour, and when it's complete, Oliver is given his pay – eight pound coins in a small plastic see-through wage pouch, and he grins with pride and satisfaction. It's gratifying to witness that as his mum, and I'm delighted for him.

Later that morning Ollie, Gracie and I take Joe to play football for his local team and let Mark have a lie-in.

It's turned into a bright, crisp day, and as it's the last Sunday of the Christmas holidays we go out for tea to a local burger restaurant that's just opened. The food's a bit greasy and nondescript and, pre-cancer, that might have irritated me – post-cancer I don't really care, and it certainly doesn't affect any of our high spirits. We reflect on how stress-free the festive break has been, considering the circumstances.

Monday 4 January

To the hospital, with the boys because they're not back at school yet, for a blood test to see if my white blood cell count is sufficient to allow me to have the next round of chemo on Wednesday. The boys chat to nurse Sanjay (Sri Lanka), before coming in with me to see the oncologist, Dr Teoh. She asks how I'm feeling, offers to help with any pain relief should I need more (I don't), and generally enquires about my physical and mental well-being. Both are fine. At the end, I ask the boys if they have any questions for her.

'How's 2016 going for you so far, Dr Teoh?' asks Ollie, which makes her laugh.

I'm in a good mood, I feel great and I'm looking forward to spring.

While we're at the hospital, my video diary episode in which I reveal I've been wearing a wig for the last few weeks, goes out on our programme and on the BBC news website. As we get back into the car, I have a quick scroll through my Twitter timeline. The reaction from people is deeply supportive. Monica at work forwards me loads of emails, too, from viewers, including this one from an NHS professional:

Dear Victoria,

As a nurse I have watched all your diaries, and just before Xmas I found a breast lump. I have had them before and they have been benign, so I am hopeful this will be too. I wept today watching your diary. I love your programme. You never shy away from difficult issues either professionally or personally.

What a beautiful woman you are.

Best wishes

Violet

I reply:

Hi Violet,

Thank you for your absolutely wonderful email. You are so very kind to get in touch.

I am sending you all the positivity in the world for your results. Please do let me know (if you don't mind) how you get on. Whatever happens, you are absolutely not alone.

Love Victoria

And later that day, she sends me this:

Dear Victoria,

Thank you for your email. I am a nurse with over thirty years' experience and have been so privileged to have met some of the most amazing people from all walks of life in my career. I have seen bravery in so many forms and am still haunted by some of the most tragic circumstances I have witnessed over the years.

Ask anyone on the front line, it's the babies and children that get to us, every time.

When I saw your promotion last week for your show today, I felt so uplifted and said to my husband how pleased I was for you that the frozen cap had worked and you had not lost your hair. I had watched your diaries and like a lot of your viewers completely respected how you were dealing with your cancer. Your first diary I said to my husband, 'That's how to deal with breast cancer, she's got it.' Honestly I thought to myself, you go girl. My husband who used to listen to you on the radio told me how great you were which is why I tuned in to your TV programme and was soon absolutely taken by it. We need someone like you to tackle the difficult questions, you ask the questions that, as a viewer, I want to. I was soon hooked by your professionalism and your programme soon became part of my day, once or twice stopping me from doing what ever I should have been doing. I'm 52, not sure how old you are but think you are in your early or mid-forties (sorry if I'm wrong,) with age comes an expectancy that we can expect to have these challenges.

Today when you took your wig off, it felt like a kick in the stomach. But your little boy was right, you couldn't tell.

You don't look any different.

Hair loss, it's awful, it's horrible . . . but it is temporary. Next Christmas your hair will be beautiful, it will shine. Beauty comes in all shades. You are a beautiful lady, your hair doesn't change that.

Me, I'll be fine, I have aunts who have had breast cancer so it's pretty normal for me. I'm not as brave as you though, if I have breast cancer I don't think I could share it in the way you have. If it comes to it I will deal with it, hopefully in the same positive way that you have.

Sometimes, no matter how many hugs I give my patients, no matter how hard I try to reassure them, sometimes, I know I don't reach them. You are not a nurse or a doctor, but you have touched so many people. Please keep doing your diary, it means an awful lot to a lot of people.

And finally . . . please keep doing what your doing, keep a little back for you and your loved ones . . . professionally, we have needed someone like you for so long. Stay positive, beautiful woman.

I'll be watching you tomorrow.

Best wishes

Violet

I'm astounded by how open and candid a complete stranger is being with me. I feel profoundly privileged, and her words give me even more strength.

Tuesday 5 January

Heading into work wearing a wig, now that my colleagues know I'm wearing a wig, is a relief and yet I'm also apprehensive. Will I mention it, to break the ice, as soon as I walk in? That's what I normally do when there's a potentially awkward or embarrassing issue. Sometimes it works, sometimes it doesn't.

I say hi to everyone, and over the course of the morning several colleagues come up to me and tell me they watched the latest video diary and found it very moving.

'Be honest, did you know I've been wearing this thing for the last few weeks?' Most people say they didn't – and I think I believe them. *Think* I do. I joke with some of the team who didn't have a clue – 'Call yourself a journalist?!'

Coverage of my diary has featured in today's *Telegraph*, *Daily Mail*, *Daily Express*, the *Sun* and the *Mirror*, which concludes its leader column like this: 'By removing a wig and admitting she finds hair loss hard to cope with, Victoria's courage may help others deal with the downsides of chemo and give them strength by showing they are not alone. The BBC has its critics, but this is public service broadcasting at its very best.'

Straight after the programme, I record the podcast for the

cancer charity Maggie's. Being back in an intimate radio studio is like putting on warm slippers: familiar, cosy, delightful. With a pair of fat headphones on, concentrating on listening to what the guests are saying is a pleasure, even though the subject matter is tough – cancer and how isolating it can be. I realise I do take comfort from talking to people who are prepared to open up about their feelings on cancer.

Tomorrow is my next chemo session. It occurs to me at night that they seem to be speeding by.

Wednesday 6 January

It's the morning of the fourth cycle, and I'm eager to get started because by midday I'll be two-thirds of the way through, and finally I can see a time when this will all be over. I catch myself as I reflect on the fact that I'm buoyant, elated even, just before I sit for several hours with a freezing, tight cap of rubber on my head while toxic drugs are pumped into me. It's all relative, I suppose. Mark nips over to Tesco to get some shopping.

It's a new drug today – Docetaxel – so we'll see how that affects me.

Nurses Emma, Sanjay and Sue are cheery and sociable as always as I arrive punctually at 9 a.m. Emma makes her usual joke about Mark being obsessed with supermarket shopping.

It turns out my blood test, which was taken on Monday, showed my white blood cell count wasn't high enough, which technically means I shouldn't be having chemo today. I am momentarily hugely disappointed – I want to get on with this – but Emma tells me not to worry, and simply takes another sample, tests it and ta da! I have enough white blood cells to proceed.

Wearing the cold cap today isn't straightforward. As it begins to freeze, I seem to shrink physically as I curl my body up and try to get into the foetal position to keep warm on the armchair. Even with my vast blanket I can't get comfortable or raise my body temperature. Once thirty minutes of the cap is up, Emma fixes the new drug, Docetaxel (or, to use its trade name, Taxotere), up to the drip – for some reason this is administered through a drip, not a large syringe – and it begins to infuse slowly into my veins.

After a few minutes I start to retch, unsure if it's the cap or the drug. It's grimly unpleasant, and my earlier chirpy attitude is replaced with subdued resignation.

Mr Kothari visits, and although chatting to him is a welcome distraction, I tell him I don't feel good today. We talk about how much it would cost a patient to have all this treatment for breast cancer privately – he thinks a reasonable approximation is sixty thousand pounds. Wow. Makes me love the NHS even more.

To try to keep me distracted, Mark reads out stories from today's newspapers. It does help.

In total, it takes two hours for the drip to empty its contents into my body, by which time I feel hypothermic. It's still not over – I'm expected to sit for another forty-five minutes with the cap on my head. I can't bear it. Trying to take control of the situation, I announce to Mark and Emma that 'I'm going to take this cap off with fifteen minutes to go . . . I can't do it, I can't get to the end.'

'That's like running the London Marathon and saying, do you know what, I'm going to stop twenty-five miles in,' Mark points out, which raises a small laugh from me. And I stick with it.

I *adore* the sound of the bell when the timer goes off. It isn't very loud, but it's clear and somehow defiant, and signifies freedom for another three weeks. If I could rip this cold cap off I would, but it's tight, awkward and wet as the ice inside it melts. As soon as I'm free of it I feel normal again. I know too that I will wear it next time, and the time after that, because there are only two more cycles to go, and I'm doing it because it's worth it to me, psychologically, to have some hair.

Emma packs up my five syringes to boost my immunity and a couple of steroid tablets and we leave.

Monica forwards me a fabulous email from a woman in Oldham called Jenny who's also going through treatment, which really cheers me up:

Hi Victoria,

My name is Jenny, I'm 44 years old and I was diagnosed with lobular breast cancer early August 2015 (on my birthday no less!).

I was diagnosed on the day of my appointment; we have a wonderful breast unit here in Oldham and they don't make you wait a week, like many primary care trusts appear to, from people's stories that I've read online.

Like you I am quite a mentally strong person and, with the love and support from my family and friends (especially my husband and sister who are both comedy geniuses and have kept me laughing), found the initial appointments, consultations, prodding, poking, naked boob shots by a young man wearing an Adidas tracksuit top, and even the surgery relatively easy to deal with.

Your regime appears to be very similar to mine with sessions at similar times too. I'm really pleased that your side effects from the FEC appear manageable; I have found mine extremely hard as the vomiting was out of control for the first, almost as bad for the second and marginally better for the third, leaving me unable even to eat or shower for 3 days and I found this also impacted on the remaining weeks till the next round in terms of recovery.

Yet every cloud has a silver lining does it not? I've felt so bad I wasn't too bothered about losing my hair, it was never my crowning glory anyway, not like your gorgeous locks, Victoria; and I've discovered that my head's a lovely little shape to boot!

I believe I'm due a new round of nicknames from the hubby soon. So far I've had 'big tit, little tit', 'Collina', 'Orc' and 'Smeigle' – ha! (I know you'll get the northern humour).

I had my first Taxotere yesterday expecting the worst but so far bit tired and a wee bit blotchy but seem to be tolerating this much better; hope it lasts.

Hope your 4th goes well – I'll be thinking of you and reading your updates.

By the way the wig looks fantastic! You look fantastic!

Lots of love,

Jenny Hulston x

After such a wretched session of chemo, Jenny cannot know how comforted and cheery I feel after reading her words. Yet again the kindness of strangers is overwhelming.

Sleeping is difficult. I'm awake for a couple of hours in the night and as I'm hot, I decide to go downstairs and take my temperature, but it's not above the danger limit.

Friday 8 January

I feel really quite OK today. Taking one anti-sickness tablet in the morning helps, as does taking Gracie out for a walk before going back to bed about lunchtime. Picking up Joe from school, one of the mums tells me she wants to 'give me a thumbs up for what you're doing'.

Saturday 9 January

Severe aches around my abdomen, like an extreme period pain, wake me. I spend most of the day in bed as I can't get rid of them.

Sunday 10 January

I feel like a very, very old woman. I can barely move, am totally wiped out and find it difficult to get out of bed even to go to the loo because of agonising pains in my stomach and lower back. Mark advises me to stay where I am and says he'll take care of everything. I feel guilty but relieved.

As I drift in and out of sleep I'm aware of the front door closing, Oliver's voice, Gracie's barks and the children's footsteps.

I have zero energy, and aches in my legs and hips which remind me of going into labour. Maybe this is the cumulative effect of chemo. Despite paracetamol, Anadin and ibuprofen, I can't alleviate the aching, nor can I get comfortable in bed. Later I slowly shuffle downstairs for a bowl of cornflakes, and then walk painfully back up to bed. This is what Docetaxel does to you: whacks you sideways when you think you've been doing OK and the end is in sight.

It's the worst day I've had since I got cancer, and I hate it.

Monday 11 January

I'm still wiped out. I wake to a text from Louisa saying that David Bowie is dead. He had cancer. Selfishly I don't want to know any more and switch my phone off.

I'm in and out of sleep all day until about five in the afternoon, when I try to get up to eat something. I can barely walk because of the pain, and as a result I'm in a foul mood. I make it to the kitchen in my dressing gown, but I shouldn't have bothered; I'm so grumpy and vile I upset everyone by yelling at Mark for feeding the children what I think are too big portions of the cottage pie he's just spent an hour and a half making.

'No wonder we're all fat,' I shout offensively, not to mention inaccurately.

Mark's cross, and tells me firmly to go back to bed. I hate myself. I hate feeling shit. I hate being in a rotten mood. I hate having no energy. I hate the waste of the days. But most of all, I hate this indulgent self-pity.

The boys come up to our bedroom later and, holding back tears, I apologise over and over again. They are pretty blasé about my horrid behaviour earlier, and very forgiving.

From hearing the news on the radio, both children have registered that David Bowie had cancer. They ask about his death and what kind of cancer killed him. I force myself to read about him. Bowie didn't tell anyone he was ill. I explain to the children that he was a smoker, but I tell them I don't know if that's what caused his cancer.

Tuesday 12 January

I hear the clock from the church opposite chime at 3 a.m., 4 a.m., 5 a.m. I find eyelashes on my pillow when I finally wake at eight-ish, but the fact that they're falling out barely registers because I still feel like shit. My throat is swollen, it hurts to swallow, I can't lie on either side in bed because it's so painful. I don't want to talk to anyone, nor do I want contact from anyone. My mum, Alex, Nick, Louisa, Anna, Helena and Cathy send me lovely texts asking how I am, and I'm too low even to answer. The idea right now of ever going to back to work seems a million miles away. There's a possibility of me hosting a debate with the various candidates who want to be the next president of FIFA, football's world governing body, in a few weeks. The thought of it fills me with dread, even though I want to do it – I just don't know when I'll feel well enough to revise for it.

I stay in bed all day, rise to try to eat at teatime and go back upstairs at half seven. Mark and the children are carrying on as normal, but I detest that they're seeing me like this.

Wednesday 13 January

Two in the morning, and I'm awake. A couple of hours later I go downstairs to let Gracie out and make some tea and toast. Gracie is always upbeat no matter what mood I'm in, and she has a way of softening you, however you're feeling. The boys are surprised and happy to see me when they get up at half six for school. Mark's in a good mood too – it's just me pretending to be OK.

I always think it won't be me who gets the aches and pains; it won't be me who loses my hair. And it is. Not that invincible after all.

Thursday 14 January

It's announced that Alan Rickman is dead, from cancer. In an unhysterical way I find it difficult to cope with hearing about another high-profile death from cancer. And then I feel guilt – I should be grateful because I'm still here and there are families everywhere mourning loved ones who've died from this disease.

Slowly, gradually, I'm emerging from the painful fog. Today I can stand upright and walk reasonably normally without crippling aches in the tops of my legs and hips. Now, with a little energy coming back, I need to get out in the fresh air before all my muscles seize up. After days of being confined to our bedroom, feeling the crisp January breeze on my face makes me feel deliciously awake, alert, alive. Gracie's happy to be my companion, and it's a joy to see her frolicking around with other dogs in the park, her ears clapping behind her head as she runs. It's cold, but the sun is shining and I inhale the cool air and try to forget the last few days.

Apart from anything else, it is *so boring* being in bed all day.

Friday 15 January

I keep thinking about the FIFA debate – I'm hassled about it. I don't want to do it, don't feel I can do it, but on the other hand I don't want to pull out.

Louisa rings to say it's likely to happen. *Oh God*, I think privately. And to say that Ben Zand, one of our reporters, and I have both been nominated in the Royal Television Society Awards: Ben for Young Talent of the Year, and me for Network Presenter of the Year. Normally I'd be jumping around with joy at news like this – it's such a vote of confidence in our programme, considering we've been on air for less than a year – but I'm not. It's a reflection more of my frame of mind right now, in the middle of treatment, than anything else.

She tells me the date of the awards ceremony – the evening of my last chemotherapy session, 17 February. Typical. I want to go, mostly because I've never been to the RTS Awards before, and so I tell Louisa I might ask my oncologst if I can push back the final lot of drugs a few days. I'll see; I might be embarrassed to ask her next time I see her because compared to cancer treatment, an awards ceremony doesn't seem very important.

I'm going back to work on Monday. Having only presented two programmes in six weeks, I wonder if I've forgotten how to do my job.

Saturday 16 January

Record some video diary on a chilly dog walk:

'We're on Day Eleven since the fourth session of chemotherapy, and it's definitely been the most difficult to bounce back from and the most unpleasant in terms of the side effects, I think. But anyway, I'm back to normal now. What it does mean, though, is that I'm thinking about the penultimate session, which should be a cause for optimism because that means it's nearly over; actually I'm now dreading it, which is annoying.'

Cathy texts to suggest going to the Isle of Wight for February half-term. It's due to be the last session of chemo that week, I explain – but I don't want to not go because of that. She says she'll sort another date; not to worry.

Monday 18 January

Slightly apprehensive about going into work today. I wonder if I've lost some confidence, having been out of the office for what feels like weeks and weeks and weeks. Usually I only get nerves before a big programme, such as a general election audience debate, or one featuring the leadership candidates of a political party (I've hosted four of those in recent years) – not for a fairly normal Monday-morning show.

However, what happens is what always happens – as soon

as I start broadcasting I forget the fretfulness and get on with the job.

Thursday 21 January

Twelve years ago today I gave birth to Oliver, and thinking about that day makes me feel intensely happy.

Our TV programme this morning is dominated by the outcome of an inquiry into the murder of former KGB spy Alexander Litvinenko, who was poisoned in a hotel in London. I've interviewed his widow Marina before, who's campaigned relentlessly for a public investigation to be held into his murder, and today is the day we report its conclusion – that President Putin of Russia 'probably' approved the assassination of Litvinenko.

I'm pleased to have worked four days this week, particularly when, a week ago, I was thinking work was going to be impossible. It means I'm not simply a cancer patient, I'm also still a journalist.

Pick up Mark from the train station later. He's had lunch with Mark Goodier from the production company.

'Well, how did it go?' I ask as he gets in.

'Yeah, it went OK,' he says casually.

'What's the top line?'

'The top line is – I'VE BEEN OFFERED A JOB!'

I scream with joy.

'Oh my God, you're KIDDING me! Oh that is so brilliant,

darling, oh God I can't believe it, WELL DONE. I am so ecstatic for you! Amazing,' and some happy tears run down my
face.

He explains that the job will entail him coming up with new
ideas for programmes and series to sell to the BBC and others.
It's right up Mark's street. In a twenty-five-year career at the
BBC, from Radio 1, to Radio 5 Live, the World Service and
most recently at Radio 2, he's been a one-man ideas factory –
something which is relatively unusual even for an organisation
as creative as the BBC. He's constantly thinking of new con-
cepts that would work on social media, on the radio, on TV.
At the World Service, he created the award-winning *World
Have Your Say*, which changed the way the huge World Service
audience interacted with the station; then he launched *Outside
Source* (his idea again), before coming up with the original
concept for the BBC's *100 Women* series. The new job will be
perfect.

This day can't get any better. Mark, Ollie, Joe and I go out
for tea and celebrate Oliver's birthday and Mark getting work.
We're all in fabulously animated moods.

And the Isle of Wight is on for a few days after Easter. I cannot
wait to be away with friends.

Friday 22 January

I officially have about three eyelashes left on each eye. As well as that, my eyes are swollen and therefore look small and piggy-like. Plus one of them is red and streaming. It's a triple whammy, but I don't care. Nothing can dent my mood after the news that Mark has a job. Managed to get an appointment at the GP's to get some prescription eye drops.

I hold my phone above my head to take a photo of the top of it. The image shows me for the first time how much hair I've lost. From halfway across my head, ear to ear, towards the front of the forehead there are only thin strands. Then there is some longer hair at the side of my forehead. What I mostly see, though, is the white flesh of my scalp. The hair at the back of my head, although it's thinned dramatically, is mostly there. It had better grow back. I decide I'm going to take this same shot every few weeks, so I can monitor any progress.

Into my inbox arrives a deliciously curious email from a casting company, asking if, in principle, I'd be keen on appearing in a new Channel 4 drama 'about a much-loved comedian – not based on a real person. We wanted to gauge if it would be something you'd be interested in? Of course, we appreciate it wouldn't be something you'd be able to answer without knowing more about the project, but we wanted to find out in theory if you would consider being featured, if you liked the material? The shoot dates are 8 February to 17 April, and we would need to check your availability.'

How exciting. 'In principle,' I reply, 'if you can let me have a few more details, then *yes*, and by the way, I'll be out of action for a week towards the end of February for a final session of chemotherapy and away in April for three days.' It's intriguing, and I can't wait to find out more.

At night, the boys and I prepare for Ollie's birthday disco – moving the furniture around in the sitting room, getting two disco balls with flashing lights in place and ordering the takeaway pizza. I feel quite nervous for him, and hope everyone turns up. They do – the boys arrive first, and despite being aged eleven to twelve, act as though they're quite a bit younger, leaping around and being generally daft; the girls arrive together, ask for the Wi-Fi code as soon as they walk in and stay together (including all of them trying to fit into the downstairs loo at one point), giggling, on their phones and looking about sixteen years of age. Dancing and singing doesn't really begin until after they've eaten food, and I'm surprised when everyone's up for singing happy birthday as I bring the cake in (in the shape of the yellow round-faced emoji wearing black shades) for Ollie to blow out the candles. For some reason I assumed they'd think they were too cool to join in with that. Afterwards, they all do 'Whip/Nae Nae', 'Gangnam Style' and sing along to every word of Adele's 'Hello'. Chatting to a few of the boys, Mark and I discover that they are really sweet, very polite and quite gentle. And the girls, once they settle down, are fun and confident and mostly quite sensible. It's heartening – I think our future's going to be safe in their hands.

Saturday 23 January

I'm awake, so Oliver asks if I'd like to join him on his paper round, and I do. Except that, when we reach the newsagent's, another boy has taken Oliver's set by accident, so we just go for a dog walk with Gracie instead and chew over last night's party. He considers it a success (I agree) and I'm pleased for him that he feels that.

When they all go off to watch West Ham in the afternoon, a wonderful calm descends on the house. Gracie and I have a lovely routine together when we're on our own. I potter about, often in the kitchen, tidying, working or flicking through the latest copy of *House & Garden* or *Homes & Gardens* magazine, and she settles down to sleep in her basket. After a couple of hours, she knows it's time for her second walk of the day and comes over and sits at my feet to remind me.

I also spend time today booking a holiday in the South of France for the summer, where I'm hoping some of our family and friends will be able to join us. The thought of July, post-treatment, free of cancer, I hope, fills me with joy.

Sunday 24 January

Paper round, dog walk, Joe's football game for his local club, a fairly typical busy Sunday. Joe loves us watching him play, particularly when he runs down the right, muscling opponents out of the way before scoring a delicious goal. Mark, Ollie and I cheer on the sidelines, along with the rest of the Halliford Colts parents.

However, by the afternoon, my mood begins to darken. I'm aggravated about the way I look – thin hair at random lengths that continues to get thinner surrounding, basically, a bald patch, covered even indoors by a beanie to keep me warm; a swollen face and eyes, no eyelashes. I'm irritated that I even care; normally my face is not something I spend any time thinking about.

I tell Mark I can't wait to look normal again.

Monday 25 January

I email Violet, the wonderful viewer who got in touch with me earlier this month, to let her know I've been thinking about her lots, and that I hope she and her husband are OK. I want to ask about the results of her tests on the cyst she told me about, but don't.

At my appointment with the oncologist today, I tell her how painful the after-effects of the Docetaxel have been. She questions me and listens carefully to my answers before promising to give me extra steroids, on a reduced dose, which should hopefully get me through the weekend immediately following chemo more painlessly. She thinks that after I took a steroid a day on the Thursday and Friday last time, effectively by Saturday I'd 'fallen off a cliff edge', as she puts it. She adds that most people find Docetaxel hard, which is strangely reassuring. I tell her it came as a shock, particularly as the first three sessions, although unpleasant, were not debilitating in the way the last lot have been. Dr Teoh also suggests that my eyes probably aren't infected, but they're streaming perhaps because the tear ducts are compensating for having no eyelashes.

Before I leave for the blood test, I ask, sheepishly, if it would be possible to delay my last chemo for a few days so I can go to the Royal Television Society Awards. She says, quite happily, yes.

Later I receive an email shedding more light on the Channel 4 drama in which I've been asked to 'appear'.

Hi Victoria

I am casting a four-part drama for Channel 4 which has been written by Jack Thorne, and directed by Marc Munden.

NATIONAL TREASURE (A four-part drama for Channel 4)
Director: Marc Munden (*Utopia*, *The Devil's Whore*)
Writer: Jack Thorne (*This Is England*, *The Last Panthers*)
Producer: John Chapman
Exec Producers: George Ormond and George Faber
Company: The Forge
Shoot dates: 8 February–17 April 2016 overall, with rehearsals from 18 January.
Location: Leeds and London

Here is a link to official press release: http://www.channel4.com/info/press/news/cast-confirmed-for-jack-thorne-s-4-part-drama-national-treasure

There is a scene in Episode 2 where the lead character, Paul Finchley (played by Robbie Coltrane) is being interviewed by yourself! I have attached episodes 1 and 2 for you to read. These are confidential.

We shoot mostly in Leeds with a tiny bit in London. I don't have exact shoot dates for this scene yet, but I do know it's very unlikely to shoot before 15 March.

Please have a look at the scripts and let me know if this is something that interests you. Equally, if you have any questions, please call. All my numbers are below.

Many thanks for your time.

Shaheen
(Shaheen Baig Casting)

ROBBIE COLTRANE! I interview *Robbie Coltrane*. I click on the press release.

'Robbie Coltrane, Julie Walters and Andrea Riseborough will star in . . .' I don't get any further, because I'm giddy at reading the words JULIE and WALTERS. Oh my God, I might be in a drama with Robbie Coltrane and Julie Walters. Shit. And I just have to play myself. This is such a delightful thrill.

I google Jack Thorne. He's only the guy J. K. Rowling asked to write the Harry Potter stage play. Wow.

Immediately I begin reading the scripts, and they're gripping. The story is about a well-known comedian, a 'national treasure', who's accused of historical child sexual abuse. According to the script, I interview the comedian (Robbie C.) on the radio, at the time that he's being investigated by the police. Julie Walters

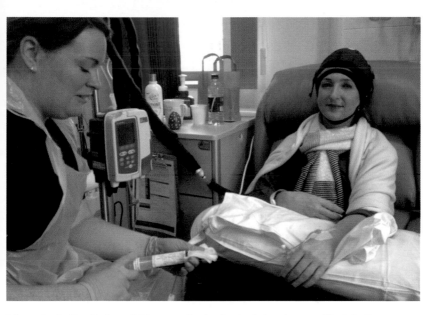

The whole family loved Emma – here she is doing her stuff while I wear a cold cap for the first time.

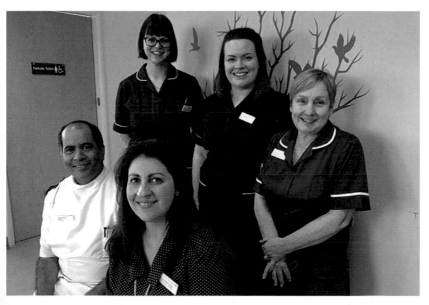

The team of nurses in the Infusion Suite at Ashford and St Peter's Hospital: *(clockwise from far left)* Sanjay, Ruth, Emma, Sue and Nicola.

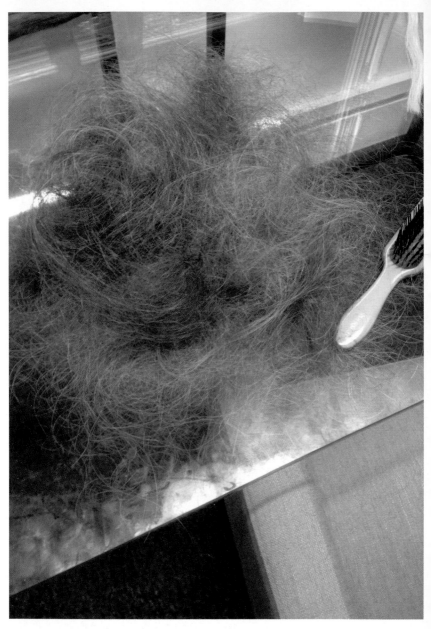

Above My hair falls out. Wigmaker Amy patiently brushed this for me.

Right From my video diary, revealing for the first time that I'd been wearing a wig. That was hard.

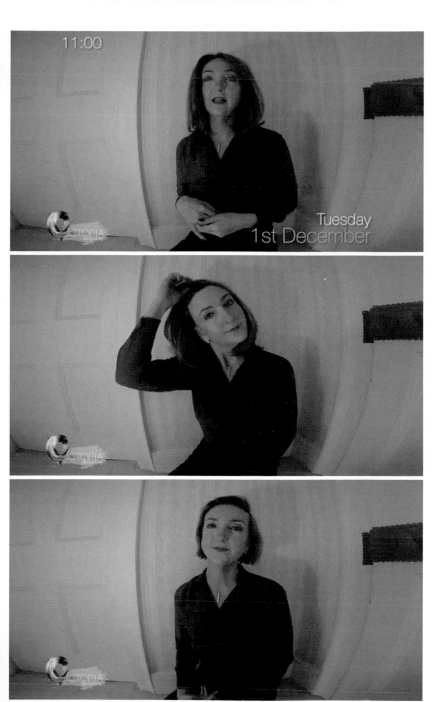

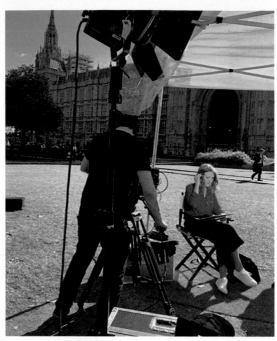

Left Presenting our programme live from Westminster.

Below My own trailer! In a car park in Leeds ahead of filming *National Treasure*.

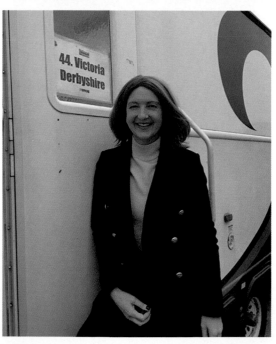

Opposite page Two acting legends and gorgeous people, Julie Walters and Robbie Coltrane.

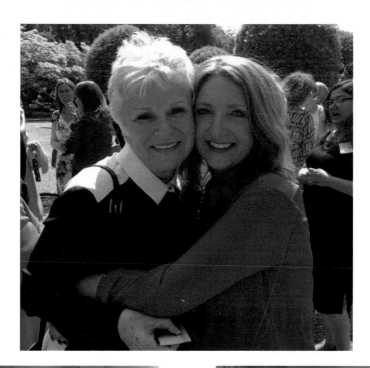

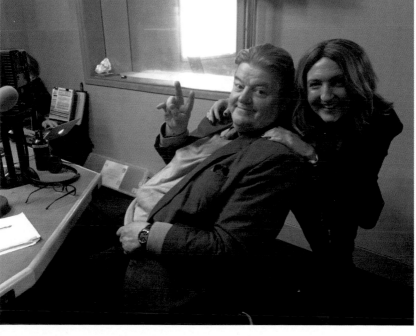

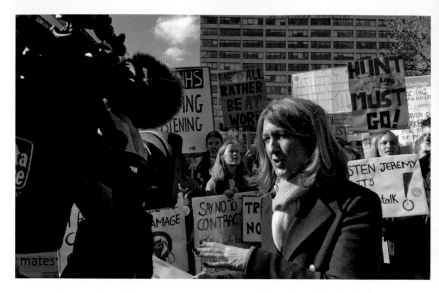

It was a huge part of my own recovery to be able to work in between chemo sessions. Here, broadcasting our programme live from a junior doctors' strike.

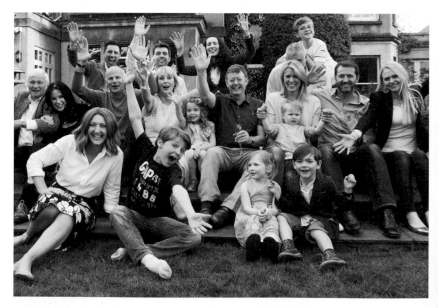

Some of my wonderful family: the photo my cousin Mark took after my relatives flew in to surprise my mum on her birthday.

This was the divine cake Mark ordered to celebrate the end of all my treatment (some of you will notice the West Ham colours).

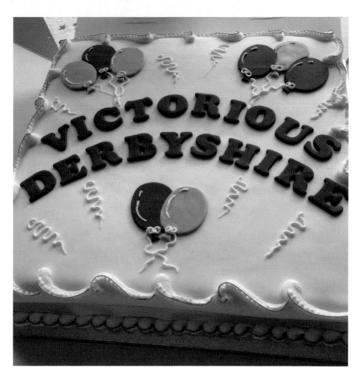

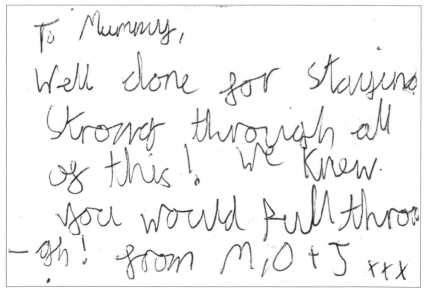

A beautiful note from Oliver, seeming more grown up than his 11 years.

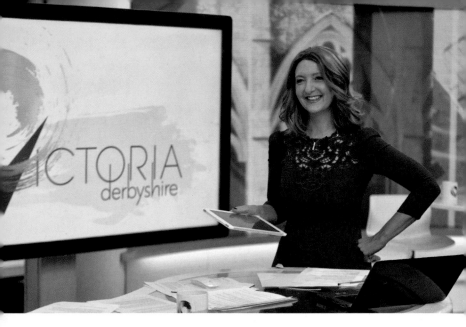

Treatment complete and back to work full time. A wig and a Dolce & Gabbana dress is a great combo. *(Geoff Overs)*

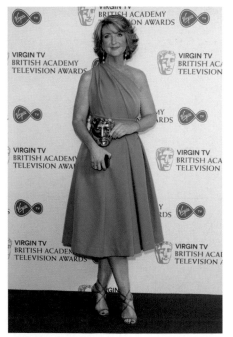

In one year I got rid of cancer and won a BAFTA TV award. Funny old world, isn't it? *(David Fisher/REX/Shutterstock)*

plays his wife and she's in the scene too. I'm going to spend time with two acting legends. How ace. I email Shaheen back and say, 'Yes, I would love to do this.'

Tuesday 26 January

At work, Louisa tells me the FIFA debate is off. It's a huge relief. Off, because the candidates are making various demands – the entourage of one says they don't want me to host the programme, while another candidate announces he won't debate with his fellow contenders. Grown men playing silly buggers.

I'm pleased to receive a reply from Violet too.

Hi Victoria,

They were benign cysts. Everything was fine, but it did make me realise after the mammogram and ultrasound etc how awful it must have been for you and how you are coping with the treatment. I thought about you all day. You have been very kind to me and I really appreciate all your positivity and concern. I was pretty sure mine were cysts but until you hear it, you always have a little doubt.

I've watched your programme and I had never really thought about it before but it made me realise that as a presenter you have to conceal your emotions just as nurses we have to. It doesn't matter what's going on in our personal life we keep everything hidden from our patients. I really don't know how you do it. You are such a positive lady.

My very best wishes for your health and happiness. I look forward to your programmes, yours are by far the best.

Thank you again for your kindness

Violet

This is what I send back to her: 'Oh, I am SOOOOOOOOOOOOOO happy for you!!!!! That is amazing news, it really is! Now go and enjoy 2016 and the rest of your life. Brilliant.'

Five months ago, my right breast collapsed. It feels like a lifetime.

Wednesday 27 January

Penultimate chemo. PENULTIMATE CHEMO. This is significant, although mine and Mark's routine is the same as it is every three weeks: I pack my chemo survival kit – blankets, a scarf, hot-water bottle and phone. Mark takes the iPad, newspapers, water and loads of bags for life so he can go to Tesco. On the car radio Chris Evans is playing 'Sir Duke' by Stevie Wonder; the words 'you can feel it all over' somehow seem appropriate ahead of what I'm about to experience in the next couple of hours.

The cold cap goes on at 9.30 a.m. and swiftly induces nausea, but again I'm not actually sick, I just retch a couple of times.

Once I get over the first fifteen minutes or so, my stomach settles down. As it's the second time I'm having Docetaxel, I'm told it shouldn't take as long as last time (two hours!) because my body will be used to it. The drugs go in without a hitch, and I close my eyes for a bit while Mark reads me some news from the paper. The drugs take one hour to infuse, just another thirty minutes with the cold cap on and we're done by 12.30 p.m. Easy.

I'm agitated in the afternoon and can't relax. I'm thinking of story ideas that we could do on our programme, and I start googling and doing some research before sending the ideas to Louisa.

The director of *National Treasure*, Marc Munden, rings to talk through what I'll be doing when we come to film the scenes I'm in in a couple of months' time. He explains why they asked me to take part; it's because the writer Jack Thorne wants the drama to be as authentic as possible, and the kind of interview I'll be doing with Robbie Coltrane's character is the kind of interview they think I would do in real life (which is true). He's friendly and impressive, and I dare to ask if it would be OK with him if I tweaked the odd word or line, because there are a couple of things in the script I wouldn't necessarily say. He's really up for that, saying Jack Thorne would want it to be as realistic as it can be, so if I could email him the changes, he'll happily run them by Jack.

I pick Ollie up from a friend's house in the evening and then take him to football training, but I'm starting to get increasingly knackered.

Saturday 30 January

Wake at 1 a.m. As I still haven't gone back to sleep by 3.15 a.m., I get up and clean the fridge.

The extra steroids Dr Teoh gave me are working, because this time three weeks ago I was in debilitating pain. There's no way I could have got up and done some housework.

Go back upstairs at half six and sit on Ollie's bed for a chat just before he gets up for his paper round.

My mum leaves a tearful message on my mobile – I'd sent her some flowers to mark the birthday of my amazing stepdad, Des. He would have been sixty-four today. He died eight years ago from a stroke, and it was catastrophic for our family, particularly my mum. I really, really, really wish he was here.

Sunday 31 January

Sir Terry Wogan is dead after a 'short but brave battle against cancer', according to a statement released by his family. I didn't know him, but met him once in the early hours at Old Broadcasting House when I was co-presenting the breakfast show on Radio 5 Live and he, the Radio 2 equivalent. He helpfully directed me to the ladies' loo, as I was unfamiliar with the building. Why does his death feel like a kick in the stomach? Because it's cancer. Again.

Monday 1 February

It's the Monday after the penultimate chemotherapy. I've spent a few days sleeping off the drugs, and am still wearily spaced out. There are about three eyelashes left on the top of each eyelid and underneath – just very, very short stubs. As a result, most of the week my eyes have been streaming. I'm actually sanguine now about any more side effects – so the eyelashes go, and I think, yep, come on, what else have you got? What else do you want to test me with?

One of our neighbours, Jak, texts to ask if we'd like a fish pie ordering from the fish man for when he comes into town on Wednesday. I say yes please, and ask how much. Another lovely gesture from one of my neighbours.

Thursday 4 February

Most of this week is spent sleeping because I'm exhausted, but I'm not experiencing excruciating pain, and for that I'm grateful.

When I open the front door to the postman, feeling slightly groggy, to sign for a parcel, there's a fish pie on the doormat, along with a note from the fishmonger, Andrew, who writes that he won't take any money for it. He says he used to love my radio programme on 5 Live and wishes me well in my recovery. I want to cry at his generosity. Meanwhile the postman asks how the treatment's going, and simply says, 'Well done.'

Mark and I go to the cinema during the day to see *Spotlight*, about the Boston Globe newspaper's investigation into child sexual abuse in the Catholic Church. It's grimly riveting. There's something cheeky about going to see a film in daylight – such a treat – and the trip out helps lift our spirits.

Friday 5 February

I sleep from 8 p.m. last night to 7 a.m. this morning.

Despite having little motivation to do anything, I'm going into town for an eyebrow tint, because as well as the eyelashes, most of my eyebrows have now fallen out, plus I'm booked in for a manicure and pedicure. On the outside I look a bugger, as my grandma used to say when she was alive, and having a bit of pampering might make me feel better about myself and my appearance. On the inside my throat is sore, my nose won't stop running and my tastebuds have become redundant. None of these things is a big deal, or insurmountable – just inconvenient. In the afternoon I eat neat peanut butter, followed by neat piccalilli and then neat Nutella, just to try to satisfy my craving for flavour. It doesn't work. I need something really spicy, I think.

Revise for a special we're doing on FIFA, corruption and the future of the organisation (without any of the candidates) on our programme a week on Monday.

Monday 8 February

I weigh myself at 4.15 a.m. I've put on half a stone since treatment began. I don't feel like I'm eating more, but clearly I'm a lot less active than normal. Plus I'm taking steroids, which can lead to weight gain. It feels pretty unimportant compared to everything else.

Back at work, and in our brightly lit studio just before we go live on air, I record some more video diary. Despite the full TV make-up, including false lashes, it can't hide my swollen eyes.

'It's thirteen days since I had the penultimate chemo session, and I'm back at work today. I'm in the studio now, and it's really good to be back and seeing everybody, and not thinking about cancer treatment or chemotherapy or side effects, and I can just concentrate on what's in the news.

'I don't know if you can see this . . . I've just noticed this on my hand [very visible on the top of my left hand are two purply-red bruised veins in a 'V' shape], which is a souvenir of chemotherapy. Those are the veins into which the chemotherapy drugs go. Anyway, that won't distract me from the programme, due to be another busy one; it can get quite intense [I walk towards the autocue] and . . . I can already see that it's the wrong day on the autocue.'

I receive a tweet from a viewer saying they could see a tear trickle down my cheek while presenting today. I explain it's not a tear in the traditional sense; my eyes are weeping simply as a side effect of the chemo.

Thursday 11 February

The sun is shining, the temperature is chilly and I'm walking Gracie.

Despite getting up at half three, or a quarter to four for the last few days, I don't feel physically tired at all. I look it; I have absolutely massive bags under my eyes, and my nose and eyes are still watering, but physically I feel all right. As Louisa says, better to look knackered but not feel it, and be alert and across stories, than look great and not be alert on air.

I've been trying to figure out why being at work at the moment is making me feel so good. I've always loved my job, but I think it's because now, more than ever, it's intensely important to my mental well-being.

Spend the rest of the afternoon reading pages and pages of briefing notes for the FIFA debate we're broadcasting in a few days, featuring former French international David Ginola; the boss of the FA, Greg Dyke; and a friend and ally of Sepp Blatter, the man who's run FIFA for decades and who is now mired in corruption allegations.

Friday 12 February

At a 9 a.m. check-up with the consultant, Mr Kothari, I ask him if, like on TV dramas, one day he will say to me, 'You're in remission.' He smiles and explains he doesn't really ever say that, but what he can tell me is that looking at the treatment I've had so far – a mastectomy and chemo – there should be no cancer in me right now. That makes complete sense to me, and seems reasonable, but still I ask if there is some blood test or some other specific method they can deploy to tell me definitively that I'm cancer-free. There isn't. He talks about the ongoing monitoring I will have – yearly mammograms on the breast that's left – but that seems so unsophisticated somehow. What I want – a diagnostic test I can take every six months, say, to tell me if cancer is present in my body – does not exist at the moment.

Saturday 13 February

In the bathroom, wearing my beanie, I'm washing my wig. It needs doing once every couple of weeks, which is a welcome change from washing my real hair every two days. It still strikes me as so incongruous, thinking about 'my wig'.

When I reflect on it, I actually can't believe I am washing a wig that I have chosen to wear because I have so little of my own hair. Anyway, it is what it is.

I take a selfie of the top of my head. For the first time I can see that new hair is growing there. Wow, and chemo hasn't even finished yet. I'm so pleased. There isn't much, just a smattering criss-crossing my scalp. Even Joe says it looks like I've got 'way more hair than Slaven Bilić now' (the West Ham manager), which makes us smile.

More prep in the afternoon for Monday's programme.

Monday 15 February

We broadcast our special on FIFA after it became engulfed in evidence of deep-seated corruption going all the way to the top man – Sepp Blatter. Because of the reading and preparation I've done, I feel in control. Paul Hayward, Chief Sports Writer for the *Telegraph*, arrives first in the green room – he looks so well after his treatment for throat cancer, which is a joy to see. We don't really have time to compare our respective treatment regimens because David Ginola strides in, just arrived on Eurostar, loud and full of energy. Then Greg Dyke and MP Damian Collins follow. Also with us is former England goalkeeper Rachel Brown-Finnis, and joining us from a studio in Freetown is Isha Johansen, who's president of the Sierra Leone FA. When I introduce Ms Johansen on air as a friend of Sepp Blatter, she immediately interrupts and says, 'The BBC always do this, always introduce me as a friend of Mr Blatter.'

'Is it not true?' I ask.

Her reply suggests it is true.

The conversation, over an hour and a half, is in-depth, comprehensive, punchy and lively, leading one viewer to comment: 'This was television journalism of the highest quality. For the first time I felt I could grasp the fundamental facts of this story.'

Wednesday 17 February

I feel stressed, and I'm not sure why.

While I'm having my make-up done in the basement of New Broadcasting House, the BBC's headquarters in London, at around 7.15 a.m., I suddenly begin to cry. It all feels too much. What, though, what feels too much? It's the last chemo next week, which I'm ecstatic about; we've got the Royal Television Society Awards tonight, which should be a good night; my family are coping brilliantly with everything (my sister says I've 'made it easy for them'); and I'm ploughing on pragmatically.

There's only me and Heather, who's doing my make-up today, in the tiny room. It's a good job, because I feel I could cry and cry and not stop. Heather gives me a huge hug.

I try and work out what's going on, and I think it's this: because I've spent the last six months focusing specifically on each part of the treatment, first the surgery, followed by each chemo cycle, I haven't allowed myself to consider the diagnosis and its impact on me. Now that this part of the treatment is drawing to a close, I'm reflecting, probably for the very first time, on what I've experienced. And I'm kind of thinking, 'What the fuck? What the fuck just happened?' It's no more profound than that.

Yet I'm conflicted too – I don't want to spend time and energy analysing it all, because I just want to get on with living.

Heather powders over the streaks on my face that the tears have created, and I carry on preparing for the programme.

I tell Louisa I'm not going to the do tonight because I just want to be at home with my boys and Mark. She spends half an hour persuading me to come, and suggests I'll probably regret it if I don't go, and she points out that it's going to be the first night out I've had in months. I relent.

Some of our team, journalists Louis, Sarah, Katie, reporter Ben, Louisa and I, meet in the Langham Hotel near work for a glass of champagne before heading to the hotel where the awards are being held. My first impressions, honestly, are that this is a vast room full of mostly white men over the age of about fifty-five. As the evening progresses, though, I see more and more journalists I admire, and I feel honoured to be nominated for such a prestigious award.

It turns out to be a great night. First of all, Ben wins his category and does a funny off-the-cuff speech (it really is off the cuff). Secondly, I'm on a table with Kirsty Wark, who's an ace journalist I respect, and not only that, she's loud and fun as well. Julie Etchingham from ITN beats Channel 4's Matt Frei and me to the Network Presenter of the Year award – which seems absolutely right, because last year she became the first woman to host one of those TV general election debates featuring various party leaders. I bump into BBC news presenter Sophie Raworth and former BBC *Breakfast* host Sian Williams, who I remember had sent Mark a kind email back in August after I was diagnosed, offering confidential support if I needed it. I ask Sian about it – which is when she reveals that she had a double mastectomy last year. I'm shocked and upset for her, and the combination of what she's sharing with me, plus alcohol, which I haven't touched for ages, means I can't help crying, albeit discreetly.

By the time I get home I can't find my keys anywhere. After

faffing around outside for about twenty minutes, I finally get in (exactly how is a secret), and decide to record a bit of my latest video diary before going to bed:

'It is just after two o'clock in the morning, and I've been to the Royal Television Society Awards for the very first time in my life, and it was a very lovely evening. We had a good laugh with our team, and Ben, who is a reporter on our programme, WON in the Young Talent category, which is brilliant. It's the first proper night out I've had in ages, as in an "out, out" night. And I must have had a good time because I have no idea where my house keys are. But obviously I've managed to get in, which is good. And in four days it's my LAST chemotherapy cycle, and . . . I . . . cannot . . . WAIT for it to be done.'

Thursday 18 February

To the hospital, for the last blood test I'll ever have before a chemo session (hopefully). At odd moments, I can't help weeping: driving to the dry cleaner's, unloading the dishwasher, sitting in the bath. Almost every time I remember that chemotherapy is coming to an end, in fact.

Sunday 21 February

In the morning, I record this: 'It's Sunday, the day before my last chemotherapy session, and I feel really relaxed, which is a contrast to the last few days, where each day for about the last four days I've shed tears, which is really unusual because I haven't cried much throughout the last six, seven months at all. And I think it's because for the whole of this process I've just been concentrating on getting through it, and taking each day as it comes as much as possible and being pragmatic and cracking on. And because it's coming to an end . . . gosh, I can feel myself getting emotional now . . . because it's coming to an end I've been reflecting on what I have experienced, and I suppose it's just a release of emotions, a release and a relief. So these are actually happy tears [smiling and pointing at a tear on my face], because it's going to be over soon.'

As the boys are getting ready for bed, I talk to each of them separately about how they're feeling. Joe says he's happy it's the last chemo tomorrow, and thinks I'll be 'euphoric' when it's over, adding it'll be 'really nice' when he gets home from school and it's all done. When I ask him how the last six or seven months have been for him, he says, 'Sometimes a bit stressful, sometimes a bit sad, but overall it's been the best it could be.' He remembers that he's had to sit a couple of lessons out because he's been worried about me, and then he closes his eyes and his face crumples into tears. My heart breaks for him; I love him so much, and feel deep guilt for putting him through this. I hug him, kiss him and tell him he's been brilliant – kind to me, compassionate, and also that he's been a strong boy.

When I ask Ollie how he is, generally, he replies, 'Yes, I'm all right, thank you,' and that the end of chemo will be 'the best thing ever, because it's going to be gone; there will be no more chemotherapy ever. Ever. Ever. It feels incredible. There have been six chemos times three weeks – that's eighteen weeks of boring, boring, boring chemo and it's rubbish. Then you can start to recover, and there will just be radiotherapy left, which is a breeze, some of your followers on Twitter say.'

I ask how the last few months have been for him.

'It's been average. There's been a lot more pressure on everyone in the family, especially Daddy, who's had to do more jobs around the house, and on you because you're wiped out for the first few days after chemo, so I'm so happy it's nearly over.'

He's being diplomatic, and I love him for that. I think he's trying to avoid saying, 'It's been really hard for all of us.'

I then ask Ollie how he thinks I've been since I was diagnosed. He thinks for a moment or two. I don't mind how he answers, but I'm nervous to hear his response. I don't want to have damaged him in any way by being ill, and I also hope to have shown him that people can cope with having cancer and come through it.

'You've been strong,' he says clearly.

I absorb his words. And respond with, 'So have you.'

Ollie smiles and adds, 'We all have.'

I thank him for being robust and pragmatic and sensible.

He says, 'And thank *you* for managing it.'

My heart bursts with pride at our thoughtful, resilient boys.

Monday 22 February

LAST CHEMO!!! Wake up at 6 a.m. in a really good mood.

Last summer I was facing the unknown, aghast at the cataclysmic news that I had cancer. Here I am today with one breast gone, little hair, no eyelashes or brows – and also, hopefully, no stray cancer cells inside me either. In a few hours' time I'll be able to put the most brutal part of treatment behind me.

Strolling down the hospital corridor following the signs to the chemo ward, I record a few thoughts on my phone: 'This is hopefully my last journey to the Infusion Suite, because today is Monday the twenty-second of February and it is my last chemo, I hope, for ever! And this is the corridor I've walked down every three weeks since November, and if I wasn't carrying so much stuff, like blankets and hot-water bottles, I would be skipping in.'

In the chair with the cap on, while the drugs are being administered and the egg timer ticking away: 'It's the last time I'm ever going to wear a cold cap, which is great – it's been a bit grim, but worth it because I've probably got about half my hair left. So yeah, that's good, I feel . . . I think I might be slightly hysterical – happy hysterical, you know – because it's coming to an end.' I wipe away tears from my eyes. 'Cos it's over soon . . . you just can't help it, really.'

Mark is with me as usual, and this is the easiest session of the six. It seems to pass quickly.

Suddenly the egg timer rings, which means it's finished. I raise both my arms and clench my fists.

'That's it,' I say, but my voice is subdued, not triumphant. 'Cool.'

Then I draw the blanket to my eyes and cover my face. The tears are coming. I can't believe it. I can't believe I've had cancer. I can't believe I've endured chemotherapy. I can't believe that's it. I'm shell-shocked.

'Well *done*,' says Mark, emphatically.

Nurse Emma walks over, because she's heard the bell.

'Did you just ding-a-ling?'

'I'm done,' I say, through smiles and tears.

Emma sings a bit of Boyz II Men: 'Now that we've come . . . to the end of the road,' as she takes off the cold cap for me for the last time.

'Are you all right?' she asks.

'Yep,' adding, 'does everyone cry at the end?' as I hear the Velcro straps on my head being undone.

'Say goodbye to your little friend,' and, 'no, not everybody, although most people do.'

Mark chips in. 'Does she not get to keep it?'

'It's all a bit overwhelming, isn't it?' Emma adds.

I swap the cold cap for the beanie and put my head in my hands. It really is over. I've done it. And I can't stop tears falling from my eyes. I'd expected to be full of energy, but it is much, much calmer than that.

As soon as the cannula is out of my left hand, I get up and Mark and I hug.

'Well done,' he says again, before adding drily, 'seems like only yesterday you were diagnosed,' which makes me laugh because we both know it's taken quite a while to get to this point. Seven months of anxiety. Seven months of uncertainty.

Seven months of tremendous highs and crushing lows.

Coat on, scarf on, bag packed, Mark offering to carry the blanket, I record one last brief bit of the video diary in the Infusion Suite, as the tears still come:

'I'm done. I'm done.'

In the car, Mark and I hold hands as I ring Cathy and tell her it's over. We both cry. I text everyone to say it's finished.

While Mark goes to collect the boys from school, I sit on my bed and reflect:

'I'm home . . . and . . . I'm happy . . . and I can't stop crying, which is mad. I think it might be six months of tears coming out in one go, if that's possible. I don't know if that's possible, or logical, or sensible, but I'm just trying to find a reason why. I think when . . . when it was over, the drugs had stopped going into me through the IV drip and the cold cap was coming off, I felt . . . in shock. I couldn't really speak, which is not like me at all, as you'll have gathered. And then I just texted my family and my close friends to say, in capital letters with three exclamation marks, 'I'M DONE!!!' [tears still streaming] So yeah . . . now I just wanna see my boys after work . . . after work? After *school*, and have a cuddle and a celebratory tea . . . and . . . get on with the rest of my life.'

Keith from work rings me to say, simply, 'Well done.' He's been a rock. And also to tell me James Harding had requested he call me to ask if I would like to present the youth EU referendum debate on BBC1 in May. I say YES immediately, and feel thrilled to be considered.

Half an hour later: 'I think I have no more tears left! I feel a little bit tired, but knowing that this is the last time I'll feel tired, four hours after chemotherapy, and that everything will be the last time, is great. And I feel a bit like . . . in your face, chemo. I really do! I've got some energy back and some feistiness back . . . and, yeah . . . goodbye chemo.'

The boys arrive back from school and shout a happy 'Hi!' as they open the front door. I'm in the kitchen making tea, and they burst in holding an enormous bunch of flowers. I scream with joy, raise my arms aloft as they cry, 'Happy end of chemo, Mummy,' and 'No more chemo,' and both give me huge hugs. Have I been happier than I feel right now? This moment is definitely up there.

Tuesday 23 February

I start to come down a little from the high of yesterday, but that's OK because *it's the last time* I'll feel like this, and psychologically that's empowering.

Mark's working in Liverpool and Salford today and tomorrow, and texts halfway through the day to say, 'Love you. I know you won't feel so good towards the end of the week but this is the beginning of a new era.' It sure is.

Take Gracie out, collect the boys from school and generally get on with things.

Wednesday 24 February

Mark's still in Salford, so I get up and take the boys to school/the station and take Gracie out for a brief walk, even though I don't feel like it at all because I'm lethargic and dehydrated.

I sleep until at about half twelve, when the cavalry arrives in the shape of Anna. She takes over, marching Gracie out for her second walk and collecting the boys when their school day is finished. It's a relief to know I can simply concentrate on sleeping and trying to get my energy back.

Thursday 25 February

Really not sure what day it is. Feel absolutely shattered, although it doesn't matter because, and I'm not going to tire of saying this, this is the last time I'll feel like this, thirty-six hours after chemo. Anna comes again in the afternoon while Mark is at work, simply because I can't physically do all the running around that needs to be done. She's a star.

Friday 26 February

All this sleeping is becoming really boring now. I'm impatient for the after-effects to be over.

Astonishingly, there is some *more* new hair growing on the top of my head. Wow.

Sunday 28 February

I'm slowly getting better. Sleeping for ten hours a night and several during the day helps, but I don't have a choice. My hair is definitely growing back – until you see confirmation of it there on the top of your head, you do actually have doubts about it regrowing. Irrational and absurd? Yes. A normal fear? Yes. And it's so dark. After twenty years of highlights, I've forgotten how naturally dark it is. I'm impatient for my eyelashes and brows to come back now too.

Wednesday 2 March

I take six bottles of champagne to the Infusion Suite to give to Emma, Ruth, Linda, Sanjay, Nicola and Sue – a team of skilled and compassionate nurses who've looked after me so well in the last few months. I don't cry, which I'm surprised about – they're all busy but spare me a few minutes to chat, and it's lovely to see them. I take some photos on my phone to remember them all, and leave. This visit feels final – like drawing a line under the treatment and the experience.

Friday 4 March

Louisa finishes editing the 'end of chemo' video diary. She's done it beautifully, as she has with all of them.

Mr Kothari asked a while ago if I'd attend a 'patient feedback' event at the hospital. It's today, and I'm really happy to go along because I want to support his ambition to expand the breast cancer unit there to make it even better for patients. Over sandwiches and cups of tea, I get to meet other women who've been treated at Ashford Hospital, too, and who are looking well, which is heartening. We spend an hour and a half talking to hospital bosses and managers, letting them know how the service there could be improved. I make sure I tell them how incredible the staff were to me – professional, kind, caring and expert. And then add, wouldn't it be amazing if they could get to the stage of letting women know their diagnosis within twenty-four or even forty-eight hours after their initial consultant appointment? Taking away the days of crippling anxiety while you wait to find out if you have cancer would be a huge step forward.

Meanwhile, there's more than a smattering of new hair on the top of my head, according to my latest 'hair selfie'. It's mostly dark, with the odd grey. The combination of the fresh short hair with the straggly longer bits which I've managed to preserve does not make for a particularly good look, but I'm simply grateful it's coming back.

Monday 7 March

From home I watch the diary of my final chemo session as it goes out on our programme today. It's as though I'm watching somebody else – this isn't me on screen enduring this, and it makes me cry. Judging by the messages I receive, it makes others shed tears too.

Tuesday 8 March

Last night's London *Evening Standard* and today's *Mirror* have similar headlines about the latest diary – 'I just "can't stop crying," says TV's Derbyshire after finishing final session of chemotherapy', and, in the tabloid, 'I'm home, I'm happy and I can't stop crying.' The *Mirror*'s leader column goes on to say this: 'BBC presenter Victoria Derbyshire's personal courage in releasing the video diaries of her treatment for cancer is an outstanding public service for women and men battling the disease.

Her honest accounts will hopefully dispel fears and give heart to people who find themselves on the same emotional health rollercoaster. We hope she's now stopped crying after completing chemotherapy because grateful viewers and well-wishers will be giving her encouraging smiles.' The tears have definitely stopped, finally.

Wednesday 9 March

I'm back to work full-time today, and it does feel very different compared to returning for just a few days at a time in between chemo sessions. There's a reassuring permanence, a welcome, drama-free normality to turning up in the newsroom. On air I choose to wear a red dress, because I feel bold and on top of the world that the harshest treatment is over and some semblance of routine is returning. I can really crack on now.

A magnificent email arrives from Richard Bacon in the States, where he's living and working at the moment. He's just seen my latest video diary, and says watching it 'feels like you're observing someone go through this privately – but you're their best mate so you've been allowed behind the curtain. In other words, you're not watching someone on TV,' adding, 'People facing chemo will look that up on YouTube for years to come and have a much better feel for the process they are about to face.'

Today feels so normal. I present the programme, and

afterwards we go and pre-record an interview for later in the week. I'm back in the old routine.

There's an email, too, in my work inbox which arrived on Monday from a literary agent asking if I'd be interested in writing a book.

Wow. I like the idea of writing a book, but I'm not a writer and there's no free time. Although what is it that's written on the clock Anna gave me a few months ago? 'There is no such thing as the right time. There is no such thing as the wrong time. There is only time.'

Monday 14 March

I take my first tamoxifen tablet today, which I will do each day for up to ten years. Some breast cancers rely on the hormone oestrogen in order to grow. This type of cancer – my type of cancer – is called oestrogen-receptor-positive. Tamoxifen blocks oestrogen from reaching the cancer cells. This means any cancer either grows more slowly or stops growing altogether; tamoxifen is therefore used after surgery to reduce the risk of breast cancer coming back. It also brings down the odds of getting a new cancer in the other breast. Two of the most common side effects of tamoxifen are hot flushes and joint pain, both of which sound OK to me.

It occurs to me that if I was still having chemo, I'd be having it today. It feels absolutely awesome not to be going through it any more. The top of my head, meanwhile, is fully covered with soft, fresh hair – there are no bald bits showing any more. It seems absurd now to think that at one point I doubted my hair would ever grow back.

Saturday 19 March

Mark and I get cross with each other for the first time in months and months over something insignificant; and the boys are going without any computer time for being poorly behaved. Yep, things are getting back to normal.

Tamoxifen, annoyingly, is causing me more trouble than I was expecting. When I wake in the morning and get out of bed, walking those first few steps is awkwardly painful – my muscles around the tops of my legs ache and click as I try to get them going again. And then all day I can feel a dull ache around my abdomen, like constant period pain. An irony, because I haven't had a period since chemo started. For a fleeting moment I think, I'm not sure I can do this for ten years. And then immediately there's a feeling of guilt – if I'm still here in ten years' time, I should be bloody grateful.

Sunday 20 March

Ollie scores a hat trick for his football team today. He's on a high, and as a result so are we.

Tuesday 22 March

I'm off work today because I have an appointment at St Luke's NHS Cancer Centre in Guildford to plan my radiotherapy timetable. It takes me about forty minutes to drive there because I get slightly lost. Walking in makes me feel unsettled and cross. I resent being here because I feel like I've put hospitals and treatment and sickness behind me, and this is like starting again.

I don't have a pass to leave my car in the car park, so the receptionist prints one out for me. It doesn't mean you get to park for free, though; it's four quid an hour.

The waiting room is vast yet claustrophobic because the ceiling is low, illuminated by strip lighting and packed full of people with cancer. Many are elderly and are wearing their own dressing gowns while waiting for radiotherapy to treat either breast or prostate cancer. I bring down the average age by about twenty years, I reckon, something that doesn't happen very often.

It strikes me as so very British: men in striped robes with their contrasting socks and shoes on, women with their pink fluffy gowns over their flesh-coloured tights and in their cosy house slippers, chatting away as though it's the most normal thing in the world to be dressed like that in public. There are three or four seating areas – big, wide blue chairs with wooden arms arranged sociably in a square around a low coffee table covered in magazines. I don't feel sociable in the slightest, so sit apart from everyone else and read some briefs for tomorrow's programme on my phone. Right in the centre is a large unfinished jigsaw puzzle of a white turreted palace on a German hillside, laid out on a table. There is no natural light, which to me makes it feel depressing. I realise I can hear the Four Tops' 'Reach Out' blaring out from somewhere.

I don't want to be here, being reminded that I have (had?) cancer.

There's a half-hour wait before meeting a member of staff called Helen (from England), who explains what radiotherapy is, which is good because I have absolutely no idea. Essentially I will lie on a large bed and above me will be a radiotherapy machine that delivers high-energy X-rays. This machine is an unwieldy, old-fashioned-looking piece of equipment that swings round like a giant pendulum to target the X-rays onto me to kill any minute cancer cells still lurking in the breast tissue.

Today is about calculating precisely where the rays need to land, by measuring angles and distances from my side to where my right breast used to be to the middle of my sternum, and so on. The aim is for the radiation to avoid as much healthy tissue as possible. For them to carry out the task accurately, I lie on a bed, top off, with my arms raised above my head, and the radiographer draws various pen marks on my skin before I'm reversed into an oncology CT scanner. None of this is unpleasant or scary. In fact, it's absolutely fascinating and rather impressive. Once the scan is finished, the radiographers place several permanent ink dots around my breast, about the size of a pinhead. They will use these marks to help get me in exactly the right position on the couch next time, ahead of my first radiotherapy session.

Radiation can make a breast implant harden. If that happens you can either leave it in, or have the implant op done again. To try to avoid both those outcomes, my oncologist is recommending a lower dose of radiation spread out over a longer period of time. Hence, thirty doses over six weeks.

The staff are incredibly friendly, and say I can bring a CD in if I like which they can play while I'm undergoing radiotherapy – which explains why I could hear the Four Tops earlier. As I leave they give me my timetable for the next month and a half. Starting on 13 April, I have to go in every weekday, including on the bank holiday in May, for an appointment that takes ten minutes. Those days stretch out ahead of me, but once this lot of treatment is completed, that should be it. *For ever*.

Thursday 24 March

James Harding and Keith take Louisa and me out for lunch. It's to toast getting through surgery and chemo, and James says some amazingly generous things about my approach to it all. I thank them profusely for their support and faith in me, in us and in our programme.

Sunday 27 March

Easter Sunday, and my mum is staying for a few days with her partner, John; Mark's dad, Bob, is visiting from Devon and Alex, Alexis and the girls come over and we have a huge family Sunday lunch which Mark cooks with Alexis helping. It's bloody marvellous! In the old days when my stepdad Des was alive, he would have done all the cooking, but Mark's taken over from him and according to Joe, he even does roast potatoes as well as Des did them.

Drinking alcohol with lunch masks the pain from the tamoxifen, which is pretty debilitating, so much so I'm actually considering stopping taking it. That would be a really big deal, but for me to think about throwing in the towel means it really is shit. Why can't pharmaceutical companies invent a drug where the side effects include losing half a stone, giving you extra energy and making your skin glow?? Later I log on to a breast cancer forum and type in 'tamoxifen' to see what others say about the drug. Some of the stories are really grim, inevitably, because if tamoxifen wasn't adversely affecting you, you probably wouldn't be on a forum, you'd just be getting on with living. Instead, women are describing how lousy they feel, how low their mood is, how unbearable the hot sweats and flushes are, how crippling the joint pain is. How it's not a panacea, and you can still die from cancer even if you're on it; it goes on and on. A couple of people do talk about having breaks from it (for a holiday or a wedding, for example), which might be a temporary solution. When I think about taking this for the next decade and coping with the pain, it demoralises me. Mark knows how severely unpleasant some days are, but his view, which he acknowledges is a selfish one, is that if it reduces the risk of breast cancer returning, then I have to take it – it's a no-brainer. I know that's logical, but having just come through some pretty brutal treatment, I don't feel ready for more pain. Not yet, anyway.

Wednesday 30 March

Take Louisa and Joanna Gosling out for lunch, to say thank you to them both for their incredible support over the last few months. Joanna has presented the programme so many times while I was off having treatment, and I'm very grateful. Louisa has been an absolute rock, always there when I needed her.

We spend a lovely couple of hours together, but inside I'm flat because of the effect tamoxifen is having on me. I just don't feel in control, whereas for much of my treatment I have felt at least some element of control, which has been incredibly important to me.

Friday 1 April

I email the oncologist, Dr Teoh, to ask again about the benefits of tamoxifen and for her view on having a short break from it. Natalie suggests acupuncture or reflexology, both of which she's tried and which have helped with the aches and pains, but I know I can't face any more needles for a while. So I decide to stop taking tamoxifen for a few weeks from today. The fact that I'm taking this decision without waiting for a reponse from Dr Teoh, with all the facts, means I feel I can't cope with this right now. And taking a decision to stop – temporarily – means I'm taking control.

At night Paul, Cathy, Steve, Vicky, Phil and Debbie come over and everyone is on good form.

Tuesday 5 April

We set off for the Isle of Wight and miss the ferry because we get stuck in roadworks on the M3 (we should have gone down the A3). Pre-cancer, this might have been a biggish deal. Post-cancer, where perspective is everything, our attitude is: no problem, we'll just book spaces online on the next one and catch that. And we do. Gracie loves sitting on the boat with the sea air blowing through her fur. Cathy, Paul, Alfie and Archie arrive at the house first, then it's us, followed by John, Juliet, their eleven-year-old boy Joe plus their cocker spaniel, Jarvis. The place that Cathy has sorted for us to stay is stunning – a large, modern glass-and-wood home which featured on *Grand Designs*.

I *love* going on holiday with my friends, and we spend the next few days taking the children and dogs for walks, visiting The Needles, which is beautiful, stopping for drinks in lovely pubs and listening to music and dancing till the early hours in the house. And Louisa turns up halfway through too!

Receive an interesting email from Dr Teoh about tamoxifen. She says taking the tablets for ten years will reduce the risk of breast cancer recurring in me to 4 to 5 per cent, down from the 11 to 12 per cent after the mastectomy, chemo and radiotherapy. Wow. That's an amazing stat. She goes on, 'and as a general rule, we'd prefer that patients don't stop for more than three months'.

OK. I decide I'm going to start taking the drug again after the BBC1 EU special at the end of May. Deal.

Meanwhile, Gracie's falling in love with Jarvis but he's not interested.

Saturday 9 April

The boys go off to watch West Ham, and I start revising all there is to know about the European Union and what difference it would make to the UK if we voted to leave.

I'm a little tired of wearing my wig now, and I feel ungrateful for saying that because it's been so crucial in helping me get through treatment while allowing me to continue working. But as my real hair is growing – there's about half an inch now – it's becoming slightly more uncomfortable.

Monday 11 April

I'm in Leeds, it's 6.15 a.m. and I'm waiting for an actor called Babou Ceesay to join me in the back of the taxi I'm sitting in. We're going to an industrial estate somewhere in the city where our hair and make-up will be transformed to help us play our roles in Channel 4's *National Treasure*. I'm playing me and Babou is playing the lawyer representing the accused comedian, a man called Paul Finchley played by Robbie Coltrane. I'm quite nervous about meeting Babou until he jumps in the cab and immediately announces that his wife used to work with Mark on his BBC World Service programme, *World Have Your Say*. Straight away I feel at ease, and we hit it off, chatting enthusiastically about his year. I ask question after question about the roles he's had – he's recently been in *Star Wars* – and it dawns on me that this guy's career trajectory is seriously on the up.

On arrival at the industrial estate we're led to our own 'trailers', and the ugliness of them cannot dampen my excitement. My own trailer! It's looks more like a shipping container than a trailer, but who cares? Inside is a small, bare, cold, unglamorous room with a chair, mirror, electric heater and rail to hang your clothes on, plus an ensuite loo and shower. But hey – it's got my name on the door, so Babou takes a picture of me in front of it, naturally. I get in, put the heater on and hang my 'costume' up. I've brought a selection of shirts I wear for work.

I sit there sending a few show-off texts to family and friends about the trailer and generally feeling apprehensive and a bit skittish. A production assistant knocks on the door at 7 a.m. and leads me in the dark to another much larger trailer, with mirrors lining the wall down one side above a shelf filled with make-up. At one end is Julie Walters in mid-conversation, so I don't say hello because I don't want to interrupt, even though my brain is shouting THAT'S JULIE WALTERS. I sit down and introduce myself to the make-up woman, who I talk to about my wig. I'm never embarrassed or shy talking to make-up pros about it because they've seen it all before.

Soon after, the trailer door opens and in climbs Robbie Coltrane. I immediately introduce myself and stretch out my hand to shake his, and tell him I'm very excited about today but also nervous because 'this is not my world'. He guffaws and says, 'Well, welcome to my world, which is full of bullshit!' It breaks the ice and we laugh and then Julie (*Julie* – I'm calling her Julie as though I know her) joins the conversation by saying it's been a long shoot and she's quite ready for it to come to an end now, but is grateful to have had two weeks at the beginning for rehearsals which, I ascertain, doesn't always happen, and which for actors makes a big difference in terms of preparing them for their role.

Then Robbie says, 'Right, shall we practise our lines?' After a second or two's silence, I realise he's talking to me, gulp conspicuously, scream inside my head 'aaaahh I've got to rehearse with Robbie Coltrane and I'm scared', but say calmly, 'Yes, sure.'

Thank God I've learned my lines.

There I am, looking in a mirror while make-up is being applied to me, with Julie Walters on my right having her make-up done and Robbie Coltrane to my left having his make-up done, rehearsing the scene we will film later. It's surreal. Sometimes I remind Robbie what his next line is. To be fair, he's got thousands to learn; I only have a few.

He's genuinely interested in whether the interview in our scene would actually happen in the real world. His character has been arrested and released on bail, so legally, I tell him, the case is known as 'active' – that is, as journalists we can't do anything that might prejudice any possible future trial; but because he hasn't been charged (yet), there's a little more leeway in what we can do. In reality, though, I say, someone being scrutinised for alleged historical child sexual offences probably wouldn't do an interview like this because they have more to lose than gain. Over the years, we've had the odd case where an individual at the centre of allegations has wanted to do an interview with me, but their lawyer's advised them not to.

At about 8 a.m. we're driven over to the BBC Radio Leeds studios in the centre of the city where our scene is being filmed. In the green room, I chat to Babou and Julie. I've recently seen *Brooklyn*, which Julie's in, so ask her about that (filmed in Montreal, it turns out, because it's cheaper than New York). At one point she says to me, 'It's so good we've got you, you know,' which embarrasses me to the point of blushing, and to which I respond, 'Oh, well, thank you, you don't have to say that at all, you know, but that's very kind of you.'

'No, no, when they said we've got Victoria we were so pleased.'

She chuckles when I tell her not to be disappointed in me

because I *am* going to ask her for a selfie before I leave today.

Next we head over to the studio, where Robbie is already sitting on his side of the 'desk' – the radio desk where there are myriad dials, faders and buttons. I meet the director, Marc Munden, for the first time, who tells me that Jack Thorne is very happy with all the amendments I made to the script. *Phew*, I think.

I sit in the 'control seat' in front of the mixing desk and Robbie and I chat away as Marc, the camera operators, script prompter and make-up and hair personnel all crowd into the studio. It's packed.

Robbie asks about my health (he knows I'm being treated for cancer, which amazes me), about where I stand on anonymity for those accused of sexual offences, which we debate quite fiercely, and I ask about his career and family and tell him my kids love him in the Harry Potter films.

And then the director actually says 'action' and I want to laugh, but as soon as we begin speaking our lines, I take it really seriously and start to feel in the zone – as though this is real and I'm genuinely interviewing a famous national figure who's accused of historical rape. It's one of the issues of our times, and the blurring of make-believe and reality in the script – this fictional character being interviewed by me, who does journalism for a living, talking about real people who've been accused of similar crimes – is clever.

Every now and then Marc interjects, recommending a particular tone for a line either Robbie or myself is saying, or to remind us of the context of what the character is thinking. We don't film it all in one go; we say a few lines and then a camera position will change, or Marc will want us to say a phrase slightly differently.

And we film the whole scene in total perhaps six to eight times. The thrust of the argument put forward by Robbie's character, Paul Finchley, is that because Jimmy Savile was never caught and prosecuted before he died, the police are trying to make up for that monumental failing by going after other high-profile men in the public eye.

As the interviewer, I point out that for every innocent man investigated, like Paul Gambaccini, there are also guilty men – Rolf Harris, Stuart Hall – and that Savile simply forced the police to go out and catch abusers.

The director wants the latter half of the scene to be quick-fire verbal jousting, and I know that's exactly how it would be if this was an interview genuinely taking place on our programme.

EPISODE 2, SCENE 11

INT. CONTROL ROOM. RADIO STATION – DAY 5

MARIE (Julie Walters) and JEROME (Babou Ceesay) standing behind mixing desks watching PAUL FINCHLEY (Robbie Coltrane) being interviewed by VICTORIA DERBYSHIRE.

PAUL: This is all wrong. I want them to police my case — I want them to prove me innocent — and I want the likes of Rolf, Stuart, Jimmy caught. But not like this.

VICTORIA: What's the alternative?

PAUL: Conduct the case in private, of course.

VICTORIA: But the police argue that by

publicising names it encourages other women who
may also have been abused to come forward. This
was crucial in the cases of Stuart Hall, Rolf
Harris and Max Clifford.
(*knowing*)
We don't know the details of your case, of
course.

There's a pause. PAUL shoots a dangerous look
at his lawyer JEROME.

PAUL: I — can't — disclose—

VICTORIA: Of course you can't.
(she looks up and meets his eyes)

VICTORIA (CONT'D): I suppose the question
is what the law should be doing. Protecting
possible victims or protecting possible
perpetrators. What do you say, Mr Finchley?

*We pull back out behind the glass as Paul
flounders.*

JEROME and MARIE watch — their faces falling.

And there the scene ends.

At one point Robbie appears to have forgotten his lines, which
leads the script lady to prompt him.

'That was meant to be a dramatic pause,' he says drily.

It takes about four hours to film this three-minute scene, and
I love every second of it. Before I leave I have selfies with Robbie
and Julie, and then I'm done. The stars and the crew have been

incredibly professional as well as warm and friendly. I feel very lucky to have been asked to be involved, and to have spent the morning with two acting legends. Everyone thanks me, but I thank them more.

Wednesday 13 April

Mark starts his new job at Wise Buddah today, and I have my first radiotherapy session. It's miles away – twenty-one there and twenty-one back to my house. The appointment is at 1.40 p.m. (I've requested half one-ish because it allows me time to get back from work in central London, pick up the car, head over to Guildford and drive back to collect Joe from school at 3 p.m.). I'm seen at around ten past two and whip my top off and lie on the bed, which rises up at the press of a button. The radiographers (two plus a trainee) line me up precisely, matching the measurements they took the other week, instruct me not to move at all and leave the room before switching the main strip lights off and the machine on. It swings ponderously above and over me, emitting its rays onto the right-hand side of my chest (you can't see them; it's not like a *Star Wars* light sabre). It's completely painless, and is over in ten minutes. I'm slightly stressed only because I'm wondering if I'll get to Joe's school in time. I do. If this session is anything to go by, radiotherapy's easy, but the travelling to and from the clinic every day, five days a week for six weeks – an hour's round trip – is going to be a total pain. They don't do radiotherapy at my local hospital, but hopefully one day they will, for other patients. Anyway, at least radiotherapy has started, and it means that in six weeks I can draw a line under the major treatment.

Mark fills me in on his day when he gets home – he likes the people, the office, the environment. After all the caring he's done for me in the past few months, I'm happy that he's happy.

Thursday 14 April

Getting up at 3.45 a.m., presenting the programme, racing out of the BBC when it ends at 11 a.m., getting home at about half twelve, taking Gracie out for a quick walk, then driving to Guildford – today getting caught in gridlocked traffic on the A3 because of an accident – is stressful. I come off the dual carriage-way to try to make my way through the centre of the town to get to St Luke's, but that's jammed too. I ring Mark, upset and cross, to announce that this is not sustainable and I'm not going to do it every day. He advises me to turn round and go home, and in the meantime he'll try to think of a solution. Not long after I've collected Joe from school, radiographer Helen calls me from St Luke's to find out why I didn't arrive for my appointment today. A bit sheepishly I explain what happened (I'm now thinking I gave up on the journey too easily for something that's so important). Helen says we'll need to find another day to fit in the dose from today.

Friday 15 April

Feel shattered, like I've been punched in the face. It's a combination of the after-effects of chemo, getting up early for work and travelling, I think.

Mark suggests I email Dr Teoh to ask if it's possible to switch the radiotherapy to a hospital in central London, so I could get there more easily straight after work. I suspect I know the answer, but it's worth a try.

At night we hold a party to celebrate the first anniversary of our programme. Twelve months ago we launched our TV news and current affairs show and I had little idea the year would include such highs and lows. Louisa and I meet early to have a drink and a catch-up in the downstairs bar where the party's being held, at which point James Harding walks in. I burst out laughing because it looks like the worst-attended do ever.

It's a brilliant night. I love our team so much.

Check my emails on the train on the way home – Dr Teoh says if I wanted to have radiotherapy elsewhere I'd have to start from scratch, leading to a delay of three to four weeks, and as I've already started, 'a gap isn't ideal'. I knew it would be a no, but at least I've tried.

Sunday 17 April

It's my mum's birthday, and she's down for the weekend along with John, her sister – my auntie Angela – and Angela's bloke, Tony. My mum has no idea that her and Angela's brother, Kevin, who lives in New Zealand, has arranged to fly in to see her on his way back from Las Vegas. Plus we've also secretly invited our cousin Mark Connor, my mum's godson, who also celebrates his birthday today. I adore surprises.

When Mark and Caroline arrive with their two little children, my mum is absolutely delighted to see them. Half an hour later, Kevin and his wife Karen walk in with a big bunch of flowers and say, 'Is there a party round here?' It's magnificent, and my mum is so stunned she can barely speak. Along with Katie, Nick and their son Max, Alex and Alexis and their girls, we all head over to the local pub for a meal before going back to the house for birthday cake and speeches. It's the kind of big family gathering that happens only once in a while, and I feel very grateful to be here and part of it.

Mark (Connor) takes a brilliant photo of us all for posterity.

Monday 18 April

Travelling a forty-odd-mile round trip for a ten-minute appointment is quite frustrating; presumably it's an issue for hundreds and hundreds of patients – you cannot always get the bespoke treatment you need at your local NHS hospital. There's absolutely nothing anyone can do about it, though, so you simply have to put up with it.

Wednesday 20 April

Victoria Wood dies from cancer, aged sixty-two. Oh, God. No one can believe it. I went to her old school, Bury Grammar, and most of us former pupils feel really proud that she became one of the funniest women in Britain (although I doubt it had much to do with school). It's a shock – only her family, it seems, knew she had cancer. But sixty-two? Come on. Enough, enough now.

Thursday 21 April

The Queen celebrates her ninetieth birthday today, and it dominates our programme.

At radiotherapy, I ask the staff if it would be OK to film the machine twisting around me while I'm lying on the bed in the radiotherapy room, and they say yes. I've previously emailed their manager to check it would be OK. Filming it gives me another purpose – I'm not simply there as a cancer patient, I'm there as a reporter. Helen tells me she's watched back the first video I did after the mastectomy and says she was impressed I was filming the day after the op. 'The day *of* the op! I think I was on a high because of the drugs.' 'Great drugs, then,' she jokes. Six down, twenty-four doses of radiotherapy to go. That's still a lot. So far, no side effects, though, so that's a positive.

Later I drive to see Amy in Richmond because my wig needs a slight repair. I talk to her about a hair system I've heard about called Intralace™, which might be useful for me while my hair's growing back. Essentially, from what I understand, a mesh cap is placed securely over your hair, which is very gently pulled through the cap, and then hair extensions are attached to the cap. Once it's on, you can do all your normal activities – like go swimming on holiday, wash and dry it as you usually would, and so on. Plus it doesn't stop your hair growing underneath. The only thing that puts me off is having to go back to the salon every six to eight weeks for them to maintain it. Amy tells me she has clients who talk about my wig-wearing as an inspiration – I've made it OK to wear a wig, apparently. Who'd have thought.

Friday 22 April

Revise at home for a mini-debate we're doing on Monday about free speech on university campuses.

A stunning bouquet of dusky pink, cream and plum-coloured roses arrives from, er, Naomi Campbell (or more likely, her people). The card says, 'Huge apologies, love Naomi'. She was in London recently and had agreed to do a pre-recorded interview with us. We'd worked out a time that suited her and also fitted around a radiotherapy appointment. In the end, the interview was cancelled, hence the flowers and the note of apology, I guess. The roses look divine on my kitchen table, but honestly, they needn't have gone to so much trouble. Stuff like this doesn't matter one iota (a new perspective for me since cancer), and hopefully I'll be able to invite her onto our programme another time.

Saturday 23 April

Nip into work to write scripts and questions for Monday's programme on free speech.

Tuesday 26 April

Today we broadcast live from a picket line outside St Thomas' Hospital in London for two hours as junior doctors go on strike again. It's an in-depth exploration of the reasons for striking – there are a number of them, and not all to do with the introduction of a new contract – with all the unpredictability a live two-hour broadcast can bring (random supporters in fancy dress, and so on). There's passion, reasoned argument, frustration and resignation from those we interview – junior doctors, other medical professionals, patients and MPs – who are pro and anti the strike action.

Wednesday 27 April

Nine radiotherapy sessions down, twenty-one to go.

Several relatives of those who died at Hillsborough appear on the programme today, after an inquest jury ruled yesterday that the ninety-six fans who were killed died because of police errors – mistakes which for years some had tried to cover up, blaming the supporters instead. Dignity in the face of such horror, an injustice which has gone on for twenty-seven years, you rarely see – but these family members are composed and moderate and all the more powerful as a result.

I race out of the building to get home and take Gracie out before radiotherapy.

Video diary:

'I've just got back from work and I'm squeezing in a dog walk before I have to go off to the hospital again. [Gracie! Gracie! Where's your ball? Where is it? . . . Bring me your ball!] So I've dashed back from work, quick dog walk with Gracie, then I'll dash to the hospital, and when I've finished today's radiotherapy session I will be a third of the way through. It's interesting how many people don't know what radiotherapy is, including me, until I started it. It was recommended for me after my mastectomy, seven months ago, and my understanding is that when you remove the breast cancer cells, it can be difficult to remove all of them – so radiotherapy, or radiation, will kill any of those cancer cells that are still hanging around on the mastectomy site, if that makes sense. Possible side effects from radiotherapy include burning of the skin, rawness of the skin, helped if you keep the area moisturised, and also tiredness. When I asked the lovely radiographers why does radiotherapy make you tired, they said because while the radiation is killing your cells, your body is expending a lot of energy trying to repair those cells.'

Right now I'm not sure I feel any more tired than I normally do.

Thursday 28 April

Work on EU stuff at home before heading off to radiotherapy. I resent the tyranny of the daily appointments: the drive, the waiting to park because it's so busy, the business of passing time before the staff call me in, the claustrophobia of the waiting room with the low ceiling. Yet because you see mostly the same members of staff each day, you do get to know a little about their lives and jobs, which I enjoy. Helen tells me that radiographers sometimes feel unloved because no one really knows what their job involves. I ask what drew her to this kind of work, and she says simply that she was interested in this area of treatment and knew she wanted direct contact with patients. She must have made a difference to thousands and thousands of people's lives.

Saturday 30 April

We spend a fun afternoon at Helen and Stuart's with Tim and Nicky – friends from our Radio 5 Live days who we see several times a year and have such a laugh with. Conversations include how we're planning to vote in the EU referendum, our kids, cancer and MS, which Nicky was diagnosed with several years ago.

At night I start to feel flat, as though my spirit has deserted me. The only option is to go to bed early, so as not to bring Mark and the boys down, and get plenty of sleep.

Sunday 1 May

There's a dark shadow shrouding my mind when I wake up. Waves of fear and doubt engulf me, and tears fill my eyes every hour or so.

Video diary:

'Very unusually, I'm having a real wobble today. I don't know why, but I'm just thinking about – and I'm sure this is completely normal and everybody who's ever had a cancer diagnosis will think this – what if this cancer comes back? Obviously I never, ever want that to happen; I never want to go through chemotherapy again, ever. I just do not want it to come back. I don't know why this is in my head today, I don't know what the reason is, I can't think of anything rational . . . but it's there. I just want this to have been a blip, and then I just get on with my life, my kids' lives, my partner's, my family's, you know, the future . . . but I can't.'

I spend most of the day feeling edgy, restless; I don't share what I'm thinking with Mark, and try to keep out of everyone's way so my unhappiness doesn't affect the day. Wish I could find some peace.

Tuesday 3 May

There's nothing like work to distract me from bleak thoughts. During the programme today, while interviewing several parents about their decision to pull their children out of school and boycott SATS tests, I can see that one six-year-old boy looks a little upset and uncomfortable in his chair. I ask him openly what the matter is and he whispers that he desperately needs the loo, so there's nothing for it but to take him. 'Right, come on then, let's go to the loo,' I say, before asking the other guests to carry on talking while I accompany Kai off set. They look stupefied for a second, laugh nervously and, fair play to them, carry on discussing the issue.

Wednesday 4 May

After work, it's the usual dash to radiotherapy.

Friday 6 May

Waking up to sunlight makes a huge difference to my mood, helping to banish oppressive thoughts about the cancer returning. As I apply a bit of make-up before taking the boys to school and the train station, I notice in the mirror that my eyelashes and eyebrows are growing back, not exactly with gusto, but growing back nevertheless. My eyebrows are now . . . patchy, when not so long ago they were non-existent. My lashes are short and stubby, but that's progress. Hurray. Then it's down to more EU referendum revision.

At radiotherapy later, one of the members of staff I see regularly, Helen, who I feel I know a little now, informs me that I'm over halfway through: eighteen down, twelve to go. As I've stopped counting, it's a pleasant surprise.

The therapeutic radiographers, as they're known, are utterly charming, and seeing them each day breaks up the absolute monotony of these daily appointments.

My close friend Laurence rings at night. He's upset and just wants to talk. He explains that Rachel's sister, Sarah Corp, is very, very ill. I listen and tell him there are no words any of us can say to console him or Rachel or their family; it is just absolutely outrageous that this is happening to Sarah.

Saturday 7 May

The boys and Mark go off to meet the other lads and dads for West Ham's last-ever fixture at Upton Park before moving to the Olympic Stadium. It feels like a big day for them all. I half-jokingly suggest that unless they actively want to be featured on *Match of the Day* tonight, they probably shouldn't cry at the end of the game.

My day is a mixture of reading EU stuff, walking Gracie, doing the washing and general pottering while listening to Elbow loudly. 'New York Morning' and 'My Sad Captains' are so powerful, so intense, especially on full volume, that they lift me and make me feel like I'm properly alive: emerging from a groggy regimen with a hopeful future in front of me. I had the chance to meet Guy Garvey once, at the Sony Radio Awards. Colin Murray said he'd introduce me, but I turned him down because I'm so in awe of Guy. I told Colin I wouldn't know what to say to him. Can't believe I did that; it was quite pathetic of me. There is no way in the future I will not seize every chance, every opportunity, every *everything* that comes my way – including writing a book.

Monday 9 May

Alan arrives in the evening to cut my hair. Not trim it; to actually cut it into some sort of style. It's obviously going to be similar to a crew cut, and despite the fact that I've never had short hair, not ever in my forty-six years, I'm looking forward to this. Chopping off some of the longer strands that I managed to rescue from chemo with the help of the cold cap finally means the hair will be growing into some sort of shape, rather than a straggly mess.

I wonder for a moment what the point was, then, of all those hours (twelve, I add up) under a frozen cap, if I'm going to have the longer bits removed now? I didn't need to save any of it – I could have simply shaved it all off just before chemo began. Yet I know that keeping some of my hair helped me cope, psychologically, because it made me feel a little more in control of the treatment and its side effects, rather than the other way round.

Alan is definitely up for it, relishing the huge challenge of trying to make it look good. As he snips away and the thin strands whisper to the floor, I'm not in the slightest bit bothered, just intrigued to see what it will look like. By the time he's finished, I can see it is very, very short. Even though this is what I wanted, it's still a bit of a shock. Oliver and Joe tell me matter-of-factly I look like a boy, whereas Mark gets ten points for saying I look like Audrey Hepburn when clearly I don't. It's no more than half an inch at the sides and perhaps an inch on top – not a buzz cut, there is just a little more hair than that, but it's definitely masculine. I'm as happy as I can be with it, though, because it's a beginning – the beginning of my new hair.

Tuesday 10 May

After radiotherapy I travel back into London to record the voice-over for the first of a three-part BBC1 documentary series called *The Big C & Me*, which is being made for the Beeb by KEO Films. I watched a preview copy at the weekend and it's beautiful, touching and sometimes very sad. It follows nine British people living with cancer over the course of a year, and the access the documentary team have had is quite extraordinary: they are there when a gentle grandma is given her shock cancer diagnosis as she sits alongside her two grown-up daughters. They are there as a bluff pigeon fancier called Dominic from Yorkshire diagnosed with breast cancer tells his wife he loves her, while she bats his tenderness away with Northern non-sentimentality. I adore the script, which is written by the series producer Kate Scholefield; it's conversational, calm and concise, with no jarring clichés.

It begins like this:

'There's a community of people in Britain that's growing every day. It's big: there are two and a half million of us. You may know some of us. Perhaps you're a member yourself.

'We all have cancer.

'That's right. There are two and a half million of us living with cancer, and a thousand more will join us every day. But don't make the mistake of thinking a diagnosis is always a death sentence. Now, for the first time, at least half of us will survive. But then again, about half of us won't.

'It's time to ditch the hushed tones, the awkwardness; we want to share what's it really like to live with cancer. None of us has chosen to be here, but still . . . welcome to our world.'

The words are powerful and true. It feels important to talk about the reality of having cancer – the negatives and the positives – and it makes me even more determined to try to write about the reality of my own cancer experience, and thank the hundreds and hundreds of strangers who helped me through it.

Laurence rings at night. Sarah Corp died today aged forty-one. My heart breaks for her, for her husband, for Rachel, her sister Eli, her mum and dad. It's unjust, unfair, unbelievable. Why, in the lottery of who gets cancer, isn't Sarah one of the lucky ones? Why? There is no rationale, no logic; and there are no words to describe the pain my friends will be enduring.

Thursday 12 May

It's hard to get motivated this morning, after the news about Sarah. I send flowers to Rachel, but it seems a pretty futile gesture. I want her to know I'm thinking of her constantly.

I have to do EU revision, but can barely concentrate, followed by a trip to see Amy so she can wash my wig and blow-dry it in the way only she can. When she sees my short hair, her instinctive reaction is 'Awesome!' I don't agree with her in the slightest, but it's kind of her to say it. Then radiotherapy, which I won't complain about any more. I hate myself for having moaned. I know I'm lucky to be able to have it.

Saturday 14 May

Joe's into Michael Jackson, so Mark takes him to see *Thriller Live* today. Ollie goes into town with friends, and I watch three editions of *Daily Politics* to catch up with what's going on at Westminster.

Already I feel used to my hair this short. I need a few highlights in it because it is so dark, but I know I will definitely go to work with short hair one day. Although not this short. And three months after chemo has ended, you can finally, properly see my eyebrows and lashes again. In fact, my lashes seem longer and stronger than before, but maybe that's just wishful thinking.

Wednesday 18 May

I have only five radiotherapy sessions left – this time next week, I'll be able to draw a line under treatment. In my life, this countdown is monumental. It's a day I've longed for for months and months. When I begin taking tamoxifen again there will be the daily reminder that I've had cancer, along with the various side effects, but I'll just have to get over those, because taking a pill that is supposed to help prevent breast cancer recurring is clearly a sensible thing to do. I could be taking it for five to ten years, depending on when I go through the menopause.

I asked Dr Teoh what happens after ten years, and she explained that they haven't done trials for more than ten years yet, so there isn't evidence to show what occurs after that. It's disconcerting thinking that perhaps, in a decade's time, there's some sort of post-tamoxifen cliff edge you go over, but simultaneously there's little point in worrying unproductively about what may or may not happen after 2026.

I text Rachel to say I'm sending her strength and love.

Thursday 19 May

I spend the day deep in European Union briefing notes, bouncing emails back and forth with the BBC's EU analyst Tamara Kovacevic. She can find the answer to any and every question I have about the EU, and there's no way I could have done this much work without her, along with research carried out by Michael at Mentorn Media, the independent production company who produce *Question Time* and who are making next week's programme, 'How Should I Vote? – the EU Debate'. I am unbelievably apprehensive ahead of Thursday. I don't want to let the audience down – the young people who are travelling from across the country to take part – nor do I want to let the bosses down at work who've shown such faith in me.

Sitting at my dressing table, taking my make-up off before bed: 'Not something I'd normally get excited about, but let me just show you a close up of my eyes [I bring my camera right up to my eyes and point to my lower and upper lashes] There . . . and there . . . top row, bottom row, and my eyebrows, twelve weeks after chemotherapy – and I'd lost ALL my lashes and most of my eyebrows three months after my last session of chemotherapy, but they're back. It's true! They *do* grow back.'

Friday 20 May

Another day of revision and dog-walking, before an evening T20 cricket match between Essex and Surrey at Chelmsford with Ronnie Irani, a childhood friend of my brother's from their days playing together at Lancashire County Cricket Club. We bump into cricketing legend Graham Gooch, who's got to be one of the most affable men in sport. Engaging and warm, and the boys love him joshing with them about his, and their, football team.

Sunday 22 May

I decide I'm going to show my mastectomy scar in my next video diary. Surgery was seven months ago, and the reason I want to reveal it is because women (and some men) who have mastectomies worry about what the skin will look like after having a breast removed. Revealing my minimal scar is intended to be reassuring. I lift up my shirt with one hand while holding my phone camera in the other. 'And that is IT. Hope you can see that. That is my scar.' It's a gently curved line, the shape of a weak smile. It's mildly pink from five weeks' worth of radiation. The skin can turn pink, red or even burn. As I've had quite a low dosage spread out over a longer period, it's now salmon-coloured. But the scar itself is so thin it's barely visible, thanks to consultant Mr Kothari being so very good at his job.

Later I send another bouquet of flowers to Rachel to let her know she's in our thoughts every day.

Monday 23 May

Apart from my sitting my A levels, giving birth and helping organise the funeral and memorial for my stepdad, I can't think of a week as massive as this in my life. On Wednesday I complete all my treatment for cancer; on Thursday, I host a prime-time BBC1 debate on the issue of the decade.

Shit. In a good way.

Between now and then it's presenting my daily programme and revision, revision, revision, with three final lots of radiotherapy thrown in.

Wednesday 25 May

The sun is warming up as I drive the twenty-one miles to St Luke's Cancer Centre in Guildford for the last time. I worked out at the weekend that I've driven, in total, just over a thousand miles to this hospital and back over the last few weeks. The staff have helpfully brought forward my afternoon appointment to 8 a.m. because they know I'm travelling to Glasgow today, the venue for tomorrow's TV debate. I take in gifts of champagne and chocolates for the radiographers I've got to know on my daily trips here: Helen, Arul (India), Sabrina (London, to Portuguese parents), Erika (Philippines) and Kate (Kent). I thank them profusely. Then I have my final session of radiotherapy, I hope, for ever.

Lying on the bed, top off, looking up at the last grey ceiling I ever hope to see, the cumbersome radiotherapy machine clicks and beeps as it swings around me. I'm composed. From diagnosis to today is 301 days. In a lifetime, assuming you live a lifetime, it's just a blip. But what a blip.

Saying goodbye to the staff is emotional, but I'm so happy I can't stop smiling. Neither can they; my mood is infectious.

And then I leave.

As I stride out of the hospital, with the sun on my face, I'm breathless with excitement . . . BECAUSE IT'S OVER.

Suddenly a torrent of emotion – exhilaration and relief – wells up from deep inside me as I head to my car and start recording the last entry for my video diary:

'It's Wednesday the twenty-fifth of May, and I'm done. I'm

done. That was my last radiotherapy session . . . just finished this second . . . wow.'

My voice begins to break and my eyes fill with tears. I can't believe it. I catch my breath as I try to stop the tears flowing down my face. I am so happy. Profoundly and magnificently happy – smiling and weeping at the same time. And hopefully that is it for cancer treatment, for ever. I breathe deeply. Wow. I feel . . . elated. I feel . . . liberated. And the future is vivid.

The people who've helped me reach this point crowd my mind, and many of them work for the NHS: the diligent and charming radiographers who I've got to know over the last few weeks; the brilliant oncologist who will review my treatment in a few weeks' time; the registrars; the anaesthetists; the nurses in the chemotherapy ward who were such a laugh; the wonderful breast cancer nurse, Outra; the amazing surgeon who I go and see again in the summer and who, hopefully, will say, well, logic would dictate that you're cancer-free.

Then there are the remarkable strangers who got in touch and sent me inspiring messages. And my tremendous family and close friends – I wouldn't be here without them.

As I walk to the car park, the sky bold and blue above me, I reflect on the thousands and thousands of people still going through cancer treatment, or about to face it. I want to offer them all my love and strength. All of it. To help them just keep going.

On 31 July 2015 I was diagnosed with breast cancer. One mastectomy, six sessions of chemotherapy and thirty doses of radiotherapy later, I feel like this could be a fresh start. I know not everybody gets that opportunity, I'm completely aware of that, and so I am very grateful. Exceptionally grateful.

Huge sigh.

OK.

Pause. Smile.

It's time to crack on with the rest of my life.

Dear reader

Most days now I don't think about cancer. It's almost like a distant memory. Almost.

Those fears about it returning recede as time passes. Sometimes I can't believe it was me who had cancer.

But I did, and I'm still here.

I feel well. Pretty much like I used to. My first thought when I wake up in the morning is no longer 'cancer'. That burden has lifted, the pressure eased. And my routine is the same as it was pre-cancer: work, the school pick-up, going out, drinking wine.

So what has changed? The daily reminders include my short hair. I was apprehensive about discarding my wig and 'coming out', but needn't have been. Revealing that hair loss was worse for me than having a mastectomy on my 'time to stop wearing a wig' video, led to conversation and debate online, in newspapers, on Radio 2 and Radio 5 Live. Many cancer patients agreed. When I asked people not to judge me for declaring that, they didn't. They understood.

Other, more insignificant differences, post-cancer: I need even more sleep than I used to, and have started exercising regularly because it helps alleviate the joint pain caused by tamoxifen.

I've slightly reorganised my life, too, so I can pack more into it, like helping out with Breast Cancer Now and Cancer Research UK as well as YouCan, for whom I'm an ambassador; and writing this book – all without reducing the time I spend with Mark and the children.

Plus I try harder not to get stressed about stuff.

For a couple of months after treatment ended, I felt I might need to go and see a counsellor. I wanted to say to someone, 'What on earth just happened?' and I knew I didn't want to bore family and friends by talking to them about it. But as I began doing physical exercise, somehow it helped address the mental side of things too. Perhaps it's the endorphins; perhaps the gradual and steady strengthening of the body helps strengthen the mind.

What has cancer taught me? I wish there was something profound I could pass on to you. There isn't. You already know that the most important things in your life are your family, your friends and your health.

But there is this: perspective.

There are elements of having cancer that are shit. And compared to that, everything else is doable.

You've got a cold? I promise you, you'll be OK.

That annoying colleague at work still hasn't done what they're supposed to, and it's winding you up? It doesn't matter.

Getting your child to do their homework is like pulling teeth? It's really not the end of the world.

There's no Wi-Fi? Come ON.

Mostly it will all be fine.

I feel as though I've been given a second chance to really live. None of us knows how much time we have left. But however long it is, I'm going to take pleasure in every moment, surrounded by my boys, Mark, my family and my friends.

Finally, if I could say one thing to cancer it would be this:

Dear Cancer, you don't define me – you simply took over my life for 301 days, motivating me to talk boldly about you to anyone who would listen. And the more I shared your reality, the more diminished you became. Because talking about cancer really can help alleviate fear and despair.

love
Victoria

Messages from wonderful people I have never met (but would love to)

One thing that my cancer experience led me to realise is that there is solace to be found in the kindness of strangers. The public reaction to my story was humbling. Many got in touch to send their good wishes, to share their own experiences and to inspire me to keep going. I wanted to include just a few of those messages here as a way of saying thank you. (I wish I could have included them all.) I hope they will provide comfort to others, as they did to me.

Sent: 12 October 2015 21:58
To: Victoria
Subject: Your story has inspired me. Thank you

Hello Victoria,

Thank you so much for sharing your story.

It has come as a timely inspiration to me as only the other day, last week, I too was diagnosed with breast cancer.

I had a mix of emotions, I froze, I didn't believe it, suggesting another biopsy is done, I was scared for my little boy etc. etc. But later that day I saw myself as one of the lucky ones because the cancer has been caught early and I'll be having a mastectomy in about 4 weeks.

Seeing your video diary and hearing you talk positively about your cancer journey has given me a completely new outlook and renewed confidence in facing my imminent treatment and recovery.

Get better real fast and well done for helping me and all the other women out there to face cancer head on without the usual dread.

Look forward to seeing you on TV again.

Love, Marie D.

Sent: 12 October 2015 09:46
To: Victoria
Subject: Victoria's Diary

My mum died from breast cancer in 1992 aged 49. As I approach her age I have been fearful that I may have to face this too one day. Victoria has shown such courage in facing this adversity that I am reassured this morning in the effectiveness of the treatment now available and that can be faced confidently.

Thank you, Victoria, and very best wishes,

Lucy, Northampton

Sent: 12 October 2015 09:48
To: Victoria
Subject: Breast cancer

I had a mastectomy in 2011 and lymph nodes removed. I soon got back to playing golf and play 18 holes three times a week still. I'm in my 80s.

My best wishes for your future health and happiness.

Celia

Sent: 12 October 2015 13:57
To: Victoria
Subject: FAO Victoria Derbyshire – Cancer diary

Hi Victoria,

My name is Matthew Bates – I'm a 26-year-old lad from
Warwickshire. I've just watched an extract from your video diary
on the 1pm News and wanted to get in touch to say how brilliant I
thought it was.

Up until September 2014 I was also a journalist – albeit a
news editor at a local newspaper – but unfortunately I had to
resign after also being diagnosed with cancer. In my case it was a
rare and aggressive form of kidney cancer. I also had surgery, to
remove a four-inch tumour in my right kidney, the kidney itself,
and 11 lymph nodes.

I thought for a long, long time about writing a column for the
paper or doing a diary for our readers, but decided against it
because I didn't really have the bottle to go public with the news.
Unlike you!

So I just wanted to say well done and I hope you stick with
the diary in the future. I think it's a brilliant idea for someone in
a prominent media position to go under the spotlight and show
what it's like having cancer, but to do so in a positive light. There
are so many negative adverts on TV, or stories in newspapers etc
– which is of course understandable – but cancer IS a manageable
disease and can be used in a positive fashion.

In my case, the past 12 months have been the worst, but
weirdly also the best, of my life – I got much closer with all my

friends and family, went on a three-week holiday (something the paper would've never allowed!) and got engaged to the girl of my dreams!! So good things can come from an experience such as this!!

Good luck to you in your recovery and keep up the good work.

Matthew Bates x

* When I wrote to Matthew to ask his permission to include his name in this book, the reply I received was not from him, but from his mum and dad, telling me that Matthew died in October 2016. Although I never met Matthew, I was devastated to hear this news. He was young, engaged to be married and had his whole life ahead of him. In an effort to learn more about this amazing man, I began reading his blogs (matt-bates.co.uk) – they are searing, beautiful, honest and warm. It would be incredible if you could read them too.

Sent: 12 October 2015 18:46
To: Victoria
Subject: Thank you

Dear Victoria,

I have just watched your video diary on the BBC and felt compelled to contact you (I don't tweet).

You are so brave, and an inspiration to anyone affected by cancer.

My partner was diagnosed 4 years ago with bowel cancer, his journey was not straightforward and he has been emotionally challenged for all of that time. Today he watched you and was so inspired by your positivity, you have made such a difference. Thank you

I hope you continue to recover and that you will soon be back on the TV.

Regards and good wishes
Sandra Townsend

Sent: 12 October 2015 12:01
To: Victoria
Subject: I just want to say thank you

Hi Victoria,

I just want to say thank you so much for sharing your journey with us.

My partner has just been told he might have lymphoma, and this week it has been a rollercoaster ride for both of us, and we were feeling terrible over the weekend as we had to wait until today before any further PET / Biopsy were possible.

However, after watching your video diary, it made me feel that it's not the end of the world, even if it turns out to be a cancerous disease. Like you said, cancer is quite mysterious to most people, until we are hit by it, so thank you again for letting us know what it's all about.

Finally, I would like to take this opportunity to wish you all the best, and I wish to see you on air soon.

Edmond Siu

Sent: 12 October 2015 17:30
To: Victoria
Subject: BBC News

Dear Victoria,

I can't tell you how much I was inspired by your broadcast on today's BBC lunchtime news. I go into hospital tomorrow to have a small lump removed from my breast.

Thank you so much. Both my husband and I are grateful.

Pamela

Sent: 11 November 2015 18:31
To: Victoria
Subject: Victoria's video of 1st chemotherapy treatment

Dear Victoria,

Having just had my first treatment on November 4th for breast cancer and having to return to the hospital today with violent head pain I felt pretty dreadful and seeing the many people in hospital undergoing chemotherapy only made me feel as if I was in a parallel universe which in many ways we are.

I just wanted to thank you for sharing your experience, I came home from hospital and watched your film and I immediately felt supported. It's hard to process your thoughts when you don't feel well and not in control and having to depend on others for many things perhaps for the first time.

I too used the cold cap and experienced the same sensations, I kept saying to myself I'm saving my hair over and over to help tolerate the initial coldness. I hope it works for you too.

Many many thanks, Victoria, I am so grateful you are doing this for us and I wish you the very best. I'm sure we will come through this and life will no doubt return to a different kind of normal.

Kind wishes
Sally Stanbridge

Sent: 04 January 2016 21:16
To: Victoria
Subject: Cancer diary

I don't normally write emails to people I don't know but I felt I had to today.

My wife was diagnosed with breast cancer in March. She's found it a very difficult and traumatising experience as you can imagine. I lost my sister several years ago to it – I want to call it an awful disease I'm still so angry about it taking her away from me – but I believe now it isn't.

We have three young children and made the decision not to tell them at this stage. It's been a real journey of discovery for us both, lots of very dark days but also some very inspiring ones. We have to keep reminding ourselves that the word 'cancer' isn't an automatic death sentence, it's not an end to a life, just another part of the journey. A rich journey we embrace as life.

Watching your diaries and reading about your very candid experiences, whilst different from ours as each person's is a unique experience, has nonetheless given a huge amount of comfort. Each of us finds our own way to cope and deal with the dreaded 'C' word but reading about and listening to your journey has been so helpful. My family and I have spent many years supporting our local hospital's cancer centre raising money never expecting for one second for it to hit so close to home. Now even more I feel I can relate to the impact it has on the lives of both those diagnosed and their families.

Oddly I can also now understand why those I've met often have such a wonderful sense of humour and ability to exist and fully experience a moment. Something most of the rest of us miss as we're too busy texting or posting another meme on Facebook. I hope you can draw some strength from the knowledge that you're having a positive impact on so many people who otherwise would have to face this alone. I don't just mean those who've been diagnosed but also those like myself who struggle to understand the impact.

For me it's been a huge challenge to try and understand and support my wife as I'm autistic so have very little empathy or ability to be there for her in a way that can help her. But listening to your experiences have given me some chance of understanding, some chance of knowing what kind of things are affecting her, what things I should be paying attention to so I can help her.

Thank you.

Marco

Sent: 05 January 2016 17:10
To: Victoria
Subject: Chemo Hair Loss

Dear Victoria,

I hope that this message reaches you and finds you in good (all things being considered) health. I feel I can joke about such things as I also am fighting cancer right now. I am 17 and was diagnosed on the 6th October and started chemotherapy on the 26th and so am experiencing similar things to you at the minute. I am writing to you today for two main reasons.

First, I would like to congratulate you on your video diaries. Your positive attitude mixed with your ability to admit you are struggling with things such as your hair loss is inspiring to me. Thank you for raising awareness for cancer, and the problems that come with it such as having to deal with wigs and people's reaction to that. I lost my hair very soon after chemotherapy started, which I was aware would happen, but, as you mentioned, it was still probably the most painful thing to have to deal with throughout this. Wigs have totally changed my life, I can still continue to go to school and go out in public feeling like a normal teenager – and hopefully have many fooled!

I am also writing to ask you if there is any possibility that you could mention the Little Princess Trust in one of your videos. I am aware that this charity, which I hope you have heard of, does not directly affect you, but in looking at your Twitter page I was struck by how a young man had donated to CRUK in your name, post watching one of your videos. It just made me think that if you were to mention this charity, some people may feel generous. The Little Princess Trust is a charity which gives wigs to children and teenagers who have lost their hair to cancer and other illnesses. They have provided me with multiple wigs, which, if I am being honest, are they key reason I have managed to continue life as normally as possible. I ask that you mention them because they are sorely under funded and under recognised and I know that with the reach of your videos, people could be compelled to donate and therefore literally change someone's life.

I am aware this may not be possible, or quite simply something you do not want to do – in the end we might as well make this journey all about us while we can! In any case, I offer you my best wishes for your health in the future and hope to hear of your battle being over soon. I am just as positive that my journey may end as well as yours is to – after all I've said that I'll run a half-marathon when this is over (I put that down to chemo brain . . .).

. . . Thank you for taking the time to read this,

Izzy Docherty

* Heartbreakingly, Izzy died in June 2016. Her father consented to his daughter's email being included in this book. I will forever be grateful to this remarkable young woman for reaching out to me in a dark time.

_____

Sent: 05 January 2016 07:31
To: Victoria
Subject: Diaries

Hi Victoria,

I am due to start chemotherapy this year and I have just watched your diaries. I would like to say a big thank you, they have been a great help and comfort. I have been wondering and worrying about what to expect and your experience has helped me.

Keep up your positive attitude and good luck with the rest of your treatment and recovery.

Last thing I can honestly say is that I would not have known you were wearing a wig, it looks very natural.

Thanks,
Sunil

Sent: 06 January 2016 09:12
To: Victoria
Subject: thank you

Dear Victoria,

Thank you so so much for your video diary. My sister is going through chemotherapy for breast cancer and is finding it hard to share how she feels all the time. But your vlog has helped me understand more of what she is going through which has helped us all. She was able to say to me, just watch Victoria Derbyshire's vlog, that's how I feel and what has happened.

I wish you all the very best and will be hoping that you recover quickly. Roll on 2016 as you say!

With my best wishes and thanks,

Lisa

Sent: 07 March 2016 09:31
To: Victoria
Subject: YOU'RE AN INSPIRATION

Haven't stopped crying at your wonderful video diaries, truly inspirational. You've been so open, honest and given people a real and true insight in to what it is really like to have cancer and endure everything that comes with it. Well done, Victoria, you're amazing. Wishing you and your whole family a very long and happy life.

Best wishes,

Louise

Sent: 07 March 2016 10:15
To: Victoria
Subject: victoria's victory

Victoria, I hope you get to read this. Thank you for this morning's programme concerning your victory over cancer. I stood in my kitchen, alone, watching, with tears streaming down my face but not for the same reason that it was happening to you. Four years ago my wife was diagnosed with pancreatic cancer. Like you she underwent 14 weeks of chemotherapy over a period of 20 weeks because some weeks she was just not well enough for treatment. They had problems getting into a vein most weeks and Thursday was her hell day. But she bravely carried on in the hope and belief that she could be cured. A month after her final session she was very ill and was admitted to hospital for a week. They then sent her home and she was put onto a driver to continuously feed painkilling drugs into her. Four weeks later she died, a few days before her 77th birthday.

Seeing how bravely you went through the trauma of chemo, that awful, wonderful process, reminded me, if I needed any reminding, how brave my Josie was in that dreadful last eight months of her life. Too often, people think the bravery is in the physical hurt of the treatment but the real bravery doesn't get mentioned usually. That is, what is going on in the mind. No matter how much you try to believe it will work, there is that niggling doubt and when the treatment ends and it has not worked the word, bravery, takes on a whole new meaning.

God bless you for the bravery you have shown in making this

morning's programme. I have never met you and probably never will but I love you for this morning. Thank you.

God bless.

Peter Greenway

Sent: 26 May 2016 09:38
To: Victoria
Subject: Breast cancer diary

Dear Victoria

My husband and I have just watched your video diary on radiotherapy. All I want to say is thank you. I like you was diagnosed with lobular cancer last October and after a mastectomy and chemo am now about to start radiotherapy next week. So I feel I have been living the same journey as you and have found your video blogs inspiring and so so helpful. When things have been bad my husband always said what would Victoria do. I'm so grateful to you and will follow your recovery so please keep us updated.

Thank you and much love and strength to you too
Julia Kyprianou

Sent: 26 May 2016 09:38
To: Victoria
Subject: A true inspiration

My daughter and I have just watched Victoria on the TV, filming her radiotherapy diaries and I was so moved by her bravery, selflessness and determination. Victoria, I wish you good health and truly hope that this is it and you are indeed cancer free for the rest of your life. To film your journey to demystify the treatment for the benefit of others, when it would have been completely understandable to want to keep this area of your life private, was so brave and selfless. My daughter and I send you every good wish for a healthy future.

Sharon and Carina Thompson

Sent: 26 May 2016 09:53
To: Victoria
Subject: Thank you

Thank you for your latest video diary – so pleased you have reached the end of your treatment and with such positivity. You are truly an inspiration to me – I was diagnosed with breast cancer on 8th Dec, had op on 21st Dec – had chemo cycle 5 two days ago – one more to go! Then start radiotherapy. I empathise completely with your feelings about the possibility of cancer returning in the future – how do you ever switch off from those thoughts? I wish you all the very best – you are looking fantastic (the hair regrowth is very reassuring!) and thank you again for sharing your story especially to ladies like me who are feeling cancer is a very lonely place at times.

Tracey xx

Sent: 26 May 2016 10:07

To: Victoria

Subject: Congratulations.

Dear Victoria,

Huge congratulations on completing your chemo. You're a huge inspiration to me and my family. We're the same age, and I have a young family having had my little boy at the age of 42!

I'm at the beginning of the process having had my first chemo last wed. I'm on 4 lots of EC every three weeks then the Taxol plus Herceptin every two weeks for 4 lots I think. Like you, I'm trying the dreaded cold cap. I'm having the chemo before the mastectomy then radiotherapy maybe (not sure yet?).

I just want to send you my love and best wishes, you have put my poor mother's mind at rest a number of times while she watched your diaries, she thinks, well, Victoria did it, so can Siobhan!

Much love, here's to the best part of your life now,

Siobhan Xxx

Sent: 14 February 2017 16:09

To: Victoria

Subject: Your cancer blogs have helped a fellow northern lass

Hi Victoria,

Since your days on 5 Live I felt we had several things in common (I guess a good presenter makes everyone in the audience feel like that): Northern 'girls' happily living 'Down South', a love of sport and two wonderful sons. A few months ago I added the dreaded but ubiquitous BC to that list and am currently 1/3 of the way through chemo. I simply wanted to thank you for your cancer blogs, which I'm sure were informative for many but have been so much more than that for me – they have given me courage.

So there we have it – thanks, Victoria.

Warmest wishes,

A

Thank You

First, thank you to the NHS and the incredible consultants, nurses, oncologists, anaesthetists, registrars and radiographers who I met and was treated by. Particularly Mr Kothari, Dr Teoh and Outra – you cared for me, you helped me make the right decisions and ultimately you saved my life. I can never, ever repay you.

Thank you to the thousands of viewers and listeners who sent me strength and love. You have been utterly wonderful, and hopefully you now understand how much you helped me get through this. I feel a connection with you which will stay with me always.

Thank you to everyone who works on our programme – you are total stars – kind and compassionate, plus you kept me entertained throughout treatment with your texts and emails about work gossip.

Thank you to my friends – I haven't got loads of close friends, but the ones I have are amazing. You're truly very special human beings.

Thank you to my awesome sister, my brilliant brother and my glorious mum. I knew you'd be ace, and you were.

Thank you to Mark – you were magnificent. You looked after me, you loved me, you kept our family going. We've been through a lot – and we're still here.

Thank you to my boys – Oliver and Joe. Sensitive and resilient. I love you so much.

And Gracie – a joy in our life when we needed it most.

Helpful Links

YouCan supports young people whose lives have been impacted by cancer – you-can.org.uk. YouCan is based in the south-east of England but is now beginning to get referrals from further afield.

Breast Cancer Now is the UK's largest breast cancer research charity – breastcancernow.org

Macmillan Cancer Support can help you if you, or someone you know, is diagnosed with cancer – macmillan.org.uk or 0808 808 00 00

Little Princess Trust provides real hair wigs, for free, for children suffering from hair loss, as well as fundraising for research into childhood cancers – littleprincesses.org.uk

There's a supportive, open and kind community of followers on my facebook page – Dear Cancer, Love Victoria. We share our experiences and help others if we can, offering words of encouragement and advice.

Here are my breast cancer video diaries:

1. The Mastectomy – https://www.youtube.com/watch?v=zHuWdtlM_3U&t=9s

2. Chemotherapy Begins – https://www.youtube.com/watch?v=qSHStzxEa_4&t=132s

3. Hair Loss – https://www.youtube.com/watch?v=f4MwEQJ6jtk&t=379s

4. Final Chemo – https://www.youtube.com/watch?v=5IYLjeLXjB0

5. Radiotherapy and End of Treatment – https://www.youtube.com/watch?v=MNyK4hNnwW4&t=2s

6. Time to Stop Wearing a Wig – https://www.youtube.com/watch?v=p5XWiZ2qHLE

Acknowledgements

Writing is a whole new world to me, which is why I am very, very grateful to all who work at Trapeze, part of The Orion Publishing Group. And I mean everyone. They have guided me through with energy and loveliness. I particularly want to say a huge thank you to my brilliant editor Anna Valentine, who, as well as being both dynamic, thoughtful and full of ideas, really believed in me and this book. Her help and insight have been invaluable – plus she never put me under pressure, ever, which is one of the many reasons I thoroughly enjoyed the writing process.

Thank you too to the fantastic Anna Bowen and Helen Richardson who've also worked very hard to support this book, and to the wonderful Loulou Clark and Rabab Adams who designed the beautiful cover, which I adore.

Dear Cancer, Love Victoria wouldn't have happened if Felicity Blunt, a clever and kind literary agent at Curtis Brown, hadn't got in touch with me. She watched one of my video diaries and asked if I would consider writing. When we met towards the end of my treatment, I told her I couldn't write in the way proper authors or some of the best newspaper writers do. She said, 'you don't have to, just write as you'. I still tried to put up barriers saying, 'but I will write directly and bluntly and there might be swearing in it and not many long words'.

'Perfect,' she said.

Thank you,

Victoria